Human drug kinetics

a course of simulated experiments

Human drug kinetics

a course of simulated experiments

L Saunders

Emeritus Professor of Pharmaceutical Chemistry,
University of London

D Ingram

Medical Computing Unit, Department of Medicine,
The Medical College of St Bartholomew's Hospital,
London EC1A 7BE

S H D Jackson

Department of Clinical Pharmacology,
The Medical College of St Bartholomew's Hospital,
London EC1A 7BE

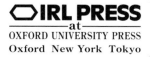

IRL PRESS
at
OXFORD UNIVERSITY PRESS
Oxford New York Tokyo

IRL Press
Eynsham
Oxford
England

British Library Cataloguing in Publication Data

Saunders, L.
  Human drug kinetics.
  1. Pharmacokinetics
  I. Title   II. Ingram, D. (David)   III. Jackson, S.H.D.
  615'.7

Library of Congress Cataloging in Publication Data

Saunders, Leonard.
  Human drug kinetics

  Bibliography: p.
  Includes index.
  1. Pharmacokinetics—Computer simulation.
  I. Ingram, D.   II. Jackson, Stephen.   III. Title.
  RM301.5.S28 1988   615'.7'0724   88-32886

ISBN 0 19 963038 0 (hardbound)
ISBN 0 19 963039 9 (hardbound plus software)

Previously announced as:
ISBN 1 85221 120 2 (hardbound)
ISBN 1 85221 121 0 (hardbound plus software)

Typeset by Design Types Ltd and Infotype Ltd and printed by Information Printing Ltd, Oxford, England.

Preface

It is a salutary fact that, despite considerable efforts of individual authors over two decades, educational computing software has tended to have a limited and rather ephemeral impact. No doubt, this has to some extent reflected early stages in a field where standards of comparison of what could be achieved were unavailable. Based on historical precedent, one should not perhaps find this surprising, given the hundreds of years from the fifteenth century which the technology of the printed word took to develop into a mature industry.

Our own involvement in the field of educational computing software spans some twenty years and in this time the computing aspect has been transformed several times over in terms of hardware and software tools and approaches. We have now reached a point where the power and flexibility is higher and where the cost of systems is lower, in relation to this performance, than could have been imagined even ten years ago.

This book and the associated software has been developed as an offering in this evolution. Our interest in the field stems from involvement over many years, in a collaboration with McMaster University Medical School, the London School of Pharmacy and St Bartholomew's Medical College. L.S. and D.I. have worked together to use the MacDope program in undergraduate courses and in research and to develop the program further for the description of human pharmacokinetics.

The program used in the present work is a completely new one designed to focus on the mechanisms of principal importance identified using the MacDope model and to provide a more streamlined and readily adaptable tool. We have been impressed by the interest taken by students, including those with limited mathematical motivation, in simulations of the type where they can design their own experiments.

In seeking to make the software more widely attractive we have linked it with a largely free-standing text which shows the scope of the program and essentially provides a course in the subject. In this way, we hope that users and teachers incorporating it in their classwork will find the program easier to use creatively than would probably be the case were we solely to issue a program manual.

We would like to express our appreciation to IRL Press for the imagination which it has shown in developing its biomedical software library. We should like to thank Paul Cullinan and Lucy Fletcher and several other readers of the text for their helpful suggestions and Duncan Daines for his help with some of the figures.

L. Saunders
D. Ingram
S. H. D. Jackson

Contents

Symbols Used in MuPharm

A	constant for biphasic equation
al	antilogarithm
al_o	old value of al
al_n	new value of al
area	area under C, t plot
$area_e$	extrapolated part of total area
$area_n$	area between 0 and t_n
$area_T$	total area to infinite time, under C, t plot
$area_{12}$	area under plot between times t_1 and t_2
α	alpha phase rate constant
b	slope of linear regression line
B	constant for biphasic equation
β	beta-phase rate constant
C	plasma concentration
C_{act}	minimum plasma level for drug activity
C_d	mean concentration in outer distribution volume
C_{leth}	minimum plasma level for lethality
C_{max}	maximum concentration
C_{mean}	mean value of C in a set of data
C_{MI}	mid-interval
C_n	concentration value at time t_n
C_S	substrate concentration
C_{SS}	steady-state concentration
C_{tox}	minimum plasma level for toxicity
C_0	value at zero time
Cl	clearance
Cl_h	clearance by hepatic route
Cl_r	clearance by renal route
Cl_T	total clearance
D	dose
D_{eo}	effective oral dose, sustained release
df( )	drug factor
ΔX_U	amount excreted in urine over a defined period
E	liver extraction ratio
E_{max}	activity when receptors are saturated
exp ( )	base of natural logs raised to power in brackets
f_i	fraction ionized (subscript o, old value; subscript n, new value)
f_{ui}	fraction unionized (subscript o, old value; subscript n, new value)
F	bioavailability
F_a	fraction of dose absorbed
F_b	fraction bound to plasma protein

F_{ion}	fraction ionized
G	fraction to first sustained release period
GFR	glomerular filtration rate
GIT	gastro-intestinal tract
h	hydrogen ion concentration
H	height in cm
i	concentration of ionized form
I	integration constant
I_1	duration of first infusion
I_2	duration of second infusion
I_D	interval between doses
k	first-order rate constant for elimination
k_a	first-order rate constant for absorption
k_d	first-order rate constant for distribution
k_m	first-order rate constant for metabolism
k_u	urinary excretion rate constant
k_o	zero-order rate constant
K_m	Michaelis constant
$\log$ ( )	logarithm to base 10
$\ln$ ( )	logarithm to base e
M	number of terms in geometric series
N	number of iterations
N_{SS}	number of doses to the steady state
P	partition coefficient, plasma to outer volume
P_u	percent of dose excreted unchanged in the urine
pH	hydrogen ion concentration exponent
pK_a	acid or base equilibrium constant exponent
rate (C)	rate of change of concentration with time
rate (X)	rate of change of amount with time
rate $(\ )_d$	rate of change due to distribution
rate $(\ )_e$	rate of change due to elimination by all routes
rate $(\ )_{form}$	rate of change due to formation
rate $(\ )_i$	rate of change due to infusion
rate $(\ )_m$	rate of change due to metabolism
rate $(\ )_u$	rate of change due to urinary excretion
rate $(\ )_{uptk}$	rate of change due to uptake from the dose
R_i	second infusion rate
RTF	renal tubular function
sf ( )	subject factor
t	time
t_I	time interval for iteration
t_{lag}	lag time
t_{max}	time at which maximum plasma concentration occurs
t_n	time of last C value in a set of C, t data
$t_{1/2}$	plasma half-life
t_{SS}	time to reach steady state

T_1	sustained release, first period
T_2	sustained release, second period
ui	concentration of unionized form
UPTK	function describing drug uptake per iteration
$UPTK_{GI}$	uptake from GIT to liver, per iteration
V	apparent volume of distribution
V_{max}	maximum rate (X) for capacity-limited process
W	body mass in kg
xd	amount in outer distribution volume
xm	amount metabolized
xp	amount in plasma
xu	amount excreted unchanged in the urine
xu_t	final value of amount excreted in the urine
X	amount of substance in mg
X_a	amount available for absorption in dosage form
X_d	amount in outer distribution volume
X_e	amount eliminated
X_{im}	amount available for absorption from i.m. depot
X_m	amount metabolized
X_{GI}	amount in GIT
X_{liv}	amount in liver
X_{rel}	cumulative amount released, sustained release
X_u	amount excreted in the urine
X_{uptk}	uptake in mg
X_o	amount absorbed from oral dose
Z	$pH - pK_a$

Introduction

This book aims to provide a course in human drug kinetics based on computer-simulated experiments. The first chapter presents an outline of the theoretical background treated in a graphical rather than a detailed mathematical form; a more mathematical treatment is given in Appendix I. Subsequent chapters contain full descriptions of simulated experiments in human pharmacokinetics. While it is preferable for the reader to be able to carry out these and other experiments, the book by itself does provide a self-contained course in the subject.

The book and the computer program together are designed to provide simulated experimental work, either as a short course in itself or as a supplement to courses in drug kinetics. The computer simulation approach is particularly useful when real practical work is difficult to arrange; it is more interesting and involving than simply working out examples with a graph and calculator, giving students the opportunity to plan their own experiments and to interpret their own results.

Educational software has sometimes failed to achieve its full potential because the authors have not demonstrated how their work can be usefully integrated within the overall teaching of the subject addressed. It is helpful to teachers for authors to show clearly the manner of use, relevance and value of their software, although the combination of writing an extensive book, in addition to a complex program, is a formidable undertaking.

In seeking to achieve this objective, the book has been planned as an account of human drug kinetics which may be used on its own but which also shows how aspects of the subject may be explored using the associated computer program, called MuPharm.

The simulated experiments are developed in a logical sequence, gradually extending the range and detail of the situations encountered. Twenty drugs, selected to cover a wide range of uses and kinetic features, are available within the program. A particular advantage is a facility whereby the user can readily add further drugs to the system.

Full details are given in the book for setting up each experiment and the reader is recommended to repeat these experiments, using his or her own machine, in order to gain familiarity with the program dialogue. Most chapters are concluded with problems on the topics covered, which are tackled by devising and running appropriate simulated experiments.

Chapters 2 and 3 are concerned with straightforward single-dose studies covering intravenous, oral and intramuscular routes of administration and designed to introduce traditional pharmacokinetic concepts and parameters such as plasma half-life, volume of distribution and clearances. The studies, which deal with a range of drugs, demonstrate how these parameters may be estimated using kinetic data.

In these two chapters, the reader is shown the procedure for setting up the experiments described and displaying the results in graphical or numerical tabular form. They therefore provide an introductory overview of the capabilities of the MuPharm program. Chapter 4 is then devoted to a full description of the dialogue which directs its operation.

Chapters 5 and 6 illustrate how clearances, and other kinetic parameters derived from single-dose experiments, may be used to design multiple-dose schedules so as to achieve mean plasma concentrations within a desired range. For this purpose each drug has defined minimum active and toxic plasma levels. With some drugs these defined levels represent a simplification of more complex plasma concentration − response relationships; the levels are, however, useful for the preliminary establishment of dosing regimens.

In Chapters 7 and 8 consideration is given to the effects of capacity-limited kinetics and of disease states on regimens and the consequent modifications required to dosing schedules.

In Chapter 9 modifications to regimens required for different subjects, particularly children and the aged, are discussed with appropriate experiments. This chapter is concluded with a set of clinical examples and problems.

The appendices may be regarded as optional extra reading. They are not necessary for using the simulation model or for courses in the subject where detail is not required. They are provided for those who would like more information on the mathematical theory and on the working of the simulation model.

Appendix I contains the mathematical basis for the kinetic relationships described in Chapter 1 and subsequently.

Appendix II summarizes properties of the twenty drugs in the simulation model.

Appendix III describes the factors used to represent different subjects in the model.

Appendix IV describes the quantitative factors used for each drug to represent the relevant drug features in the simulation model.

Appendix V outlines the overall mathematical form of the kinetic equations used in the simulation model, showing how subject and drug factors are combined in the calculations.

Appendix VI describes the setting up of a new drug file in the model, so that the drug can be loaded subsequently.

Appendix VII describes a similar procedure for setting up and storing subject characteristics.

Appendix VIII outlines the effects of changing the computational iteration interval for the calculations.

We hope that the material will be of value to a wide variety of students in medicine, pharmacy, nursing and in other health professions and medically related sciences such as medical chemistry and biophysics. Students with a limited knowledge of mathematics need not be deterred from reading the book and using the program. They will quickly learn how to use the simulation program effectively and will soon become interested in the results which it produces.

In our experience over many years, the computer simulation approach is attractive to students of widely differing aptitudes and approaches. They can make use of the resource with different levels of detail and mathematical analysis of results, according to their interests and needs.

CHAPTER 1

Drug Kinetic Theory

1. DRUG KINETICS AND THERAPEUTICS

Human pharmacokinetics involves the study of the rates of absorption, distribution, metabolism and elimination of drugs after they are given to a human subject. These rates are followed by measuring drug and metabolite concentrations in blood and urine; other body fluids, for example saliva, may also be sampled in some investigations.

The plasma concentration of a drug is one of the major factors in determining the response of the subject to that drug. A knowledge of the kinetic processes involved in establishing this concentration provides much valuable information for determining suitable dosing schedules for the drug.

Although some of the mathematics involved may appear quite complicated, it is not difficult to understand the principles involved when they are expressed in simpler terms. In this book we have adopted a primarily graphical approach to the subject; a more mathematical treatment of the theory is given in Appendix I.

The description of theoretical aspects is developed within a framework of simulated experiments with 20 drugs of widely different kinetic properties and therapeutic uses. On working through these experiments, you will see the use made of two particularly important kinetic parameters; the first is the plasma half-life of the drug which is simply the time taken for plasma concentration to halve, the second is the area under the plasma concentration–time curve.

With a knowledge of these parameters, a dosing regimen for a particular subject may be designed which will maintain plasma concentrations above the minimum level for drug activity and safely below the minimum level at which toxic effects may be expected.

In the simulation model, there are minimum values assigned for the active, toxic and lethal levels of the drug, derived from published data. The levels are readily changeable by the user to express individual subject behaviour in response to the drug. For example, as a result of drug abuse or of illness, a patient may have become tolerant to diamorphine; consequently much higher doses and plasma levels of morphine than normal are required to give significant effects. With such a patient, the active, toxic and lethal levels may be reset to appropriate values.

In this chapter, the theory of human drug kinetics is outlined in simple terms and a brief description of the simulation model is given. These two topics are treated in more detail in Appendix I and in Appendix V, which form optional extra reading, not required for understanding the development of theory in the main part of the book.

During the development of the theory reference is made to a number of drugs. The uses and particular distinguishing characteristics of these drugs are summarized in *Table 1.1*.

Only one use is listed for each drug. Most of the drugs are to be found on the main list of the simulation program; further information about them is given in Appendix II.

2. THE SOLUBILITY OF DRUGS; pH OF BIOLOGICAL FLUIDS

Most drugs are polar organic substances, polar meaning that there is a separation of electric charge within the molecule; it is this separation of charge which governs many of the physical properties of a drug, particularly the solubility.

2.1 Water-soluble drugs

A highly polar organic compound is soluble and often ionizes in water but is usually almost insoluble in lipid solvents such as ether and chloroform. For example, ampicillin and the other penicillins are so polar that a hydrogen ion readily separates from the molecule in aqueous solutions, making them quite strong acids.

Due to their insolubility in lipid solvents and in lipids, the penicillins have only a limited distribution in the body. They do not readily cross lipid cell membranes and they do not enter the body fat. They are rapidly excreted in the urine, partly because highly polar substances are not reabsorbed in the renal tubules.

2.2 Lipid-soluble drugs

Drugs of low polarity generally contain hydrocarbon groups which make them soluble in lipid solvents. In water they only ionize to a limited extent, making them weak acids or bases (e.g. digoxin). These drugs have a high volume of distribution because they are able to pass through lipid cell membranes and are able to enter the body fat. They are reabsorbed in the renal tubules and only slowly pass out in the urine.

Most drugs of low polarity are converted *in vivo* to more polar metabolites before they are excreted in the urine. In the case of paracetamol, a very weak acid, the metabolism is rapid and the plasma half-life is short.

2.3 Polar drugs with some lipid solubility

There are drugs which are both moderately polar and also have appreciable solubility in lipids. Examples are the tricyclic antidepressants such as nortriptyline, a moderately strong organic base with appreciable solubility in chloroform. Nortriptyline is strongly bound to plasma proteins and is also strongly bound outside the plasma.

As a result of these properties nortriptyline is very widely distributed in the body, showing an apparent volume of distribution much higher than the physical volume of the subject. For example, in a 70-kg male the apparent volume of distribution of nortriptyline is more than 1000 litres.

Table 1.1 Uses and characteristics of drugs in Chapter 1.

Drug	Use	Characteristics
Ampicillin	Antibiotic	Highly polar, water-soluble, strong acid, pK_a 2.5, binding 18%, partly excreted via bile, tubular secretion, incomplete i.m. absorption
Pivampicillin, Talampicillin	Antibiotics	Ampicillin esters which are pro-drugs for ampicillin
Digoxin	Treatment of heart failure (atrial fibrillation)	Low polarity, soluble in lipid, weak acid, pK_a 10
Nortriptyline	Anti-depressant	Soluble in water and lipid, 95% bound, distribution volume 1200 l, first-pass effect 50%
Temazepam	Sedative	Weak base, pK_a 1.6
Oxprenolol	Treatment of hypertension	Base, administered as hydrochloride, extensive hepatic metabolism
Phenytoin	Anti-convulsant	Acid, given as sodium salt, 93% bound, capacity-limited metabolism in the therapeutic range of doses, incomplete i.m. absorption
Theophylline	Treatment of bronchial asthma	Weak acid, pK_a 8.6, given i.v. as aminophylline, an 80% mixture with ethylene diamine
Carbamazepine	Anti-convulsant	73% Bound, enzyme inducer
Lignocaine	Treatment of arrhythmia	70% Bound, first-pass effect 65%
Diamorphine	Analgesic	35% Bound, tolerance, rapidly metabolized to morphine
Kanamycin	Antibiotic	1% Bound, relatively strong base, pK_a 7.2
Thiopentone	Short-acting anaesthetic	Biphasic $\log(C)$, t plot, alpha phase 1 h
Indomethacin	Analgesic	Biphasic, alpha phase 5 h
Salicylate	Active metabolite of aspirin	Volume of distribution, 12 l
Aspirin	Treatment of rheumatic fever	Capacity-limited metabolism in the therapeutic range
Paracetamol	Treatment of mild pain	Capacity-limited metabolism at very high doses
Phenobarbitone	Anti-convulsant	Enzyme inducer
Atenolol	Treatment of hypertension	Example for repeated doses, little hepatic metabolism
Inulin	Diagnostic agent for renal inpairment	No protein binding, no tubular absorption or secretion
Creatinine	Endogenous substance accumulates in renal impairment	No protein binding, no tubular absorption or secretion

2.4 Aqueous solubility and pH

The solubilities of weak acids and bases in an aqueous medium depend on the pH (i.e. the hydrogen ion concentration) of the medium. pH is defined as minus the logarithm to base 10 of hydrogen ion concentration. Low pH means a high hydrogen ion concentration giving an acidic medium; high pH corresponds to low hydrogen ion concentration and alkalinity of the medium. pH 7 represents acid–base neutrality and is the value for very pure water.

A weak acid, HA, is a substance which tends to donate hydrogen ions (written H_3O^+) to an aqueous medium.

$$HA + H_2O = H_3O^+ + A^-$$

If the medium is already acidic (e.g. a solution of hydrochloric acid) the ionization of the weak acid is suppressed and consequently the solubility of the weak acid is reduced, since the ionized form A^- is more soluble in water than the unionized form HA.

If the medium is alkaline (e.g. sodium hydroxide solution) ionization is promoted and the solubility is enhanced.

The opposite situation occurs with a weak base, B. A base is a substance which tends to extract hydrogen ions from water.

$$B + H_2O = BH^+ + OH^-$$

An acid medium promotes this ionization and increases the solubility of the base, while an alkaline medium suppresses ionization and decreases solubility.

The strength of an acid or base is measured by its pK_a value, a dimensionless estimate, on a log scale, of the tendency to ionize. The scale is normally from 0 to 14; for an acid, low pK_a means a relatively strong acid (e.g. ampicillin, pK_a 2.5), while high pK_a means a relatively weak acid (e.g. digoxin, pK_a 10).

For a base, the pK_a scale works in the opposite sense, high pK_a means a relatively strong base (e.g. kanamycin, pK_a 7.2), while low pK_a means a very weak base (e.g. temazepam, pK_a 1.6).

2.5 Degree of ionization, pH and pK_a

The degree of ionization of a weak acid or base is the fraction of the total concentration which is ionized. This fraction is governed by the ionizing tendency of the substance, measured by the pK_a, and the acidity or alkalinity of the medium, measured by the pH.

The degree of ionization F_{ion} is governed by the difference between pH and pK_a. *Figure 1.1* shows values of F_{ion} at varying value of $(pH - pK_a)$. The effect of this difference is in opposite directions for acids and bases.

The detail of the calculations of these values is given in Appendix I, Section 7. From the figure it is seen that if the pH of the medium is such that $(pH - pK_a)$ is outside the limits -2 to $+2$, the drug is either almost completely ionized or completely unionized.

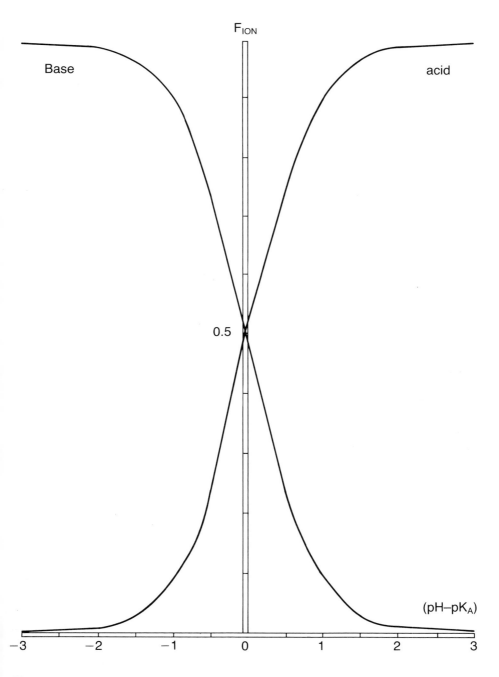

Figure 1.1 Degree of ionization and (pH − pK_a).

2.6 pH of biological fluids

2.6.1 *Blood*

The pH of arterial blood is 7.4, close to the value of 7.0 for acid–base neutrality. The blood plasma is buffered to this value by combinations of weak acids and their salts, so that it does not change appreciably when a small quantitity of a drug is added.

2.6.2 *Gastric fluid*

The lowest pH which a drug is likely to encounter *in vivo* is that of the gastric fluid, 1.0–1.5, though sometimes higher. This low pH is due to hydrochloric acid which may cause the chemical destruction of a drug such as benzylpenicillin. This drug cannot therefore be given by the oral route. The effective pH of the gastric surface at which some drug absorption may occur is around 3.5.

In the stomach the ionization of acidic drugs is suppressed; e.g. with the relatively strong acid, ampicillin, at pH 1.5, $(pH - pK_a) = 1.5 - 2.5 = -1.0$; from *Figure 1.1*, F_{ion} is less than 0.1. Weaker acids are almost completely unionized while basic drugs are completely ionized at this low pH.

2.6.3 *Intestine*

In the small intestine a drug encounters media whose pH increases progressively from that of the stomach up to 8.0, so that the degree of ionization of acidic drugs increases while that of basic drugs may decrease. The main absorption of a drug given by the oral route is in the small intestine, although slow-release formulations may continue to release drug throughout the large intestine.

2.6.4 *Urine*

The urine pH is in the range 4.5–7.5. The urine is usually acidic with a pH around 5.5. Change of urine pH can be helpful in eliminating overdoses of ionized drugs. If the drug can be further ionized by changing the urine pH, its reabsorption in the renal tubules is reduced and the rate of urinary elimination is increased.

Urine pH may be changed by administering either ammonium chloride which reduces the pH to around 4, making it more acid, or by giving sodium bicarbonate which raises the pH to around 8, making it slightly alkaline.

2.7 Degree of ionization in drug formulation

To improve absorption, drugs which are only sparingly soluble in water are often given orally as their salts. Examples are the beta-blocker oxprenolol, normally given as the hydrochloride, and phenytoin, administered as the sodium salt.

Theophylline, a weak acid of pK_a 8.6, is always, when given intravenously, administered as aminophylline, a mixture of the acid with the weak organic base ethylenediamine. This base considerably enhances the solubility of theophylline. The mixture contains about 80% theophylline. There is no clinical indication for giving aminophylline by mouth, but nevertheless it is frequently used for oral dosage.

3. PLASMA PROTEIN BINDING OF DRUGS

On entering the plasma, most drugs are rapidly bound to plasma proteins. The binding is a reversible process and the extent of binding varies with both drug and protein concentrations. For many purposes, it is the extent of binding at therapeutic levels of the drug and at normal concentrations of protein in the plasma which is of interest. This extent is expressed as the fraction bound F_b, or as a percentage, of the total drug concentration.

At high drug concentrations, saturation of the binding sites may occur, resulting in a reduction in the fraction bound. A reduction in this fraction may also be caused by displacement of the drug from the protein by another drug. Reductions in binding may be significant therapeutically if the drug has a degree of binding of 90% or more.

Protein binding incorporates the drug into a macromolecule, which is unable to cross most biological membranes. This binding would therefore appear to inhibit the wider distribution of the drug. However, a very strongly bound drug such as nortriptyline (F_b = 0.95) is also strongly attached to macromolecules and tissues outside the plasma, causing removal of most of the drug from the plasma to the outer distribution volume.

Protein binding is particularly important in the urinary excretion of unchanged drug. Only the unbound drug molecules are filtered at the glomeruli and therefore it is only the unbound fraction which is available for excretion in the urine. Drugs with a high degree of protein binding are only excreted unchanged in the urine to a very limited extent.

In general, basic drugs such as propranolol tend to bind to α_1 acid glycoprotein (AAG), whereas acid drugs such as indomethacin tend to bind to albumin. AAG is an acute phase protein, the concentration of which tends to rise during acute illnesses. This may occasionally have a detectable effect on free drug concentrations and hence alter the response to the drug as, for example, with drugs of low volume of distribution which are highly protein bound.

Some examples of degrees of binding are: nortriptyline 95%, phenytoin 93%, carbamazepine 73%, lignocaine 70%, diamorphine 35%, ampicillin 18% and kanamycin 1%.

4. KINETIC PROCESSES, ORDER, PLASMA HALF-LIFE

4.1 **Kinetic processes**

In the body a drug participates in a number of transport processes and chemical reactions. Pharmacokinetics aims to interpret these processes from experimentally measurable quantities. In human drug kinetics, these measurements are usually limited to determinations of plasma concentrations and sometimes concentrations in other body fluids such as saliva, and to estimations of amounts of the drug and its metabolites which are excreted.

The interpretations usually centre round measurements of the plasma concentration C of the drug, at times t after the dose is given. If the drug is injected rapidly into the blood as an intravenous (i.v.) bolus dose, C starts at a high value and declines with time t, as shown in *Figure 1.2*.

The rate of change of C with t decreases as time proceeds; the instantaneous rate of change at any time is measured by the slope of the tangent PR to the curve at that time. The magnitude of this slope is equal to PQ/QR, where PQR is the right-angled triangle in *Figure 1.2*.

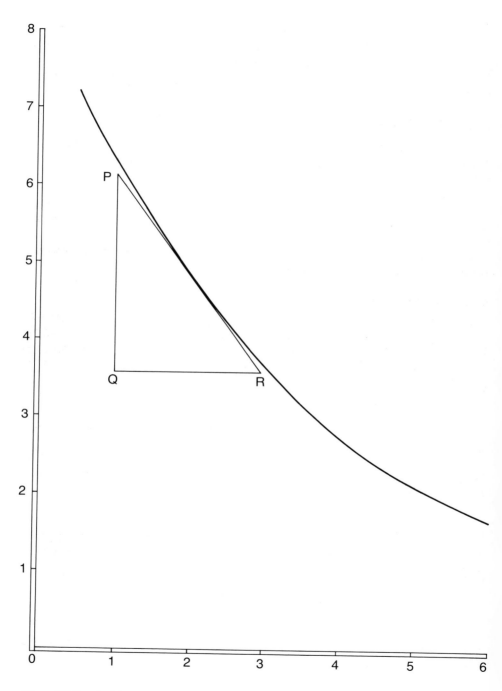

Figure 1.2 C, t plot following i.v. bolus.

The way in which the rate of change of plasma concentration, rate(C) (dC/dt in calculus notation, see Appendix I), varies with C and t is characterized by the *order* of the kinetic process. For most purposes in pharmacokinetics, it is only necessary to consider two orders, zero and first, and the combination of these two in the Michaelis–Menten equation for enzyme kinetics.

4.2 Zero-order kinetic process

A zero-order process is defined as one in which the rate is constant, independent of both C and t; the rate is often expressed as rate(X), the rate of change of amount of drug X with time, rather than as rate of change of concentration.

$$\text{rate}(X) = k_0$$

k_0 is called the *zero-order rate constant* and has the same units as rate(X), amount/time, e.g. mg/h.

In drug kinetics, an example of a zero-order process is the uptake of drug into the plasma from a constant-rate i.v. infusion.

4.3 First-order process

In this type of kinetic process the rate of change of concentration with time is directly proportional to the concentration. *Figure 1.2* is an example of first-order kinetics. While C is high the rate of change of C is rapid; as C falls the magnitude of the rate of change also falls, and the C,t curve becomes less steep. The general equation expressing first-order kinetics is:

$$\text{rate}(C) = k \times C$$

k is the *first-order rate constant*, with units (conc/time)/conc = 1/time; the units are therefore reciprocal time, e.g. h^{-1}.

In *Figure 1.2*, C decreases as t increases, the rate of change of C with t is therefore negative. In order to keep the rate constant, k, as a positive quantity, the equation for this type of process is written:

$$\text{rate}(C) = -k \times C$$

An important consequence of the first-order equation is that when it is integrated (Appendix I, Section 1.2) to give C at any time in terms of t, it is found that the logarithm of C is a linear function of t.

$$\ln(C) = \ln(C_0) - k \times t$$

$$(1.1)$$

$\ln(C_0)$ is constant, C_0 being the estimated value of C at $t = 0$ and $\ln(C)$ the natural logarithm of C; $\log(C)$ denotes the logarithm to base 10, and the two are related by

$$\ln(C) = 2.303 \times \log(C)$$

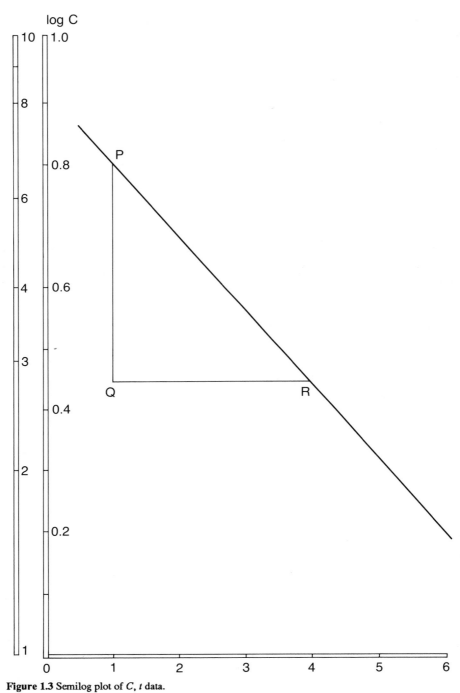

Figure 1.3 Semilog plot of *C*, *t* data.

This linear relationship between $\ln(C)$ or $\log(C)$ and t is shown by plotting the data of *Figure 1.2* as $\log(C)$ against t, when the straight line in *Figure 1.3* is obtained.

In order to obtain linear or partially linear plots, semilog graph paper is used. This graph paper has the ordinate (vertical axis) spaced according to the logarithms of numbers and the abscissa (horizontal axis) spaced arithmetically.

Semilog paper usually has logarithms to the base 10 for the spacings and the numbers shown on the ordinate (vertical) axis are values of C. The distance between 1 and 10 is the value of the log unit and is the same for any pair of values which differ by a factor of 10. The ordinate axis for semilog paper is shown to the left of the axis of $\log(C)$ in *Figure 1.3*.

The equation of the straight line in this figure is (Appendix I, Section 1.2):

$$\log(C) = \log(C_0) - (k/2.303)t$$

The slope of the line is $-k/2.303$. This plot therefore provides a method for determining the rate constant k. To do this graphically, a triangle PQR is drawn and the sides measured. Note that the length of PQ has to be in log units, i.e. the length in cm divided by the length of the log unit in cm (distance from 1 to 10 on the ordinate scale or any decade), QR is length in time units, measured along the abscissa. The magnitude of PQ/QR is then equal to $k/2.303$.

4.4 Half-life

A characteristic feature of a first-order process is that the time taken for C to decline to half its value is independent of the starting value of C, this time is the half-life $t_{1/2}$; it can be shown that $t_{1/2}$ is inversely proportional to the rate constant k (Appendix I, Section 1.3).

$$t_{1/2} = 0.693/k$$

(1.2)

Half-life is a simple concept and is generally used to characterize a first-order process.

The half-life can be found graphically from the slope of a semilog plot. It is more conveniently determined from numerical data which are known to give a linear semilog plot and therefore follow first-order kinetics. By making a regression calculation for $\ln(C)$ on t, using a programmed calculator (there is no point in using logs to base 10), the regression coefficient b, which is the slope of the best straight line through scattered points, is calculated. For a process in which $\ln(C)$ decreases as t increases

$$k = -b$$

b given by the calculator is negative, making k positive. At least three points are required for the regression calculation.

The data in *Figures 1.2* and *1.3* are for an i.v. bolus dose of 250 mg of kanamycin; the graphical estimation of k from the slope of the plot in *Figure 1.3* gives the following values:

$$PQ/QR = 0.122 \text{ h}^{-1}, \ k = 0.28 \text{ h}^{-1}, \ t_{1/2} = 2.47 \text{ h}$$

Since all the points lie on the straight line, a regression calculation is made with them all, giving the results:

$$b = -0.275 \text{ h}^{-1}, \quad k = 0.275 \text{ h}^{-1}, \quad t_{1/2} = 2.52 \text{ h}$$

5. DISTRIBUTION

5.1 Components of volume of distribution

The distribution of a drug outside the plasma is a reversible transfer of drug between the plasma and other sites, tissues and fluids in the body. The binding of a drug by plasma proteins occurs rapidly, followed by distribution to the extracellular space (fluid volume is ~11 l in a 70-kg male) and to part of the intracellular fluid (~30 l in a 70-kg male).

Further distribution through lipid membranes to the rest of the intracellular fluids and to the body fat (~10 kg in the same subject) occurs with drugs which are soluble in lipid solvents.

After an i.v. bolus dose, the drug gradually spreads out from the plasma volume into which it is injected, to the final complete volume of distribution for the particular drug.

5.2 Biphasic kinetic behaviour

The time taken to reach the complete volume of distribution for a drug may be assessed from C, t data following an i.v. bolus dose of a drug which shows first-order kinetic behaviour.

The data are plotted on semilog paper; while the drug is moving outwards from the plasma, the points lie on a curve above the late time straight line produced backwards to the ordinate axis. When the drug concentrations in the plasma and the outer distribution volume become balanced, the plot becomes linear, as is seen in *Figure 1.4*. In this figure, C_d is an estimate of the mean drug concentration in the outer distribution volume.

In human subjects detailed kinetic studies of drug distribution to individual fluids are not usually available. As a working approximation it is assumed that the outer distribution may be represented by a single mean concentration.

The type of plot shown in the upper curve of *Figure 1.4* is called *biphasic*: the *curved part* of the plot is called the *alpha phase*, the *straight line* part is the *beta phase*. All drugs show some alpha phase, which may be very brief. From *Figure 1.3* it is seen that the kanamycin plot is linear from 0.5 h, so that the complete distribution volume is penetrated in less than 0.5 h.

In Chapter 2, Section 3.3 it is shown that with thiopentone, the alpha phase lasts for about 1 h. *Figure 1.4* is for a bolus dose of 50 mg of indomethacin; the alpha phase is seen to persist for several hours.

5.3 Apparent volume of distribution, partition coefficient

Each drug is found to have its own apparent volume of distribution, ranging from 12 l in a 70-kg male for salicylate, up to over 1200 l for nortriptyline.

Polar, water-soluble, lipid-insoluble drugs have relatively small distribution volumes, while lipid-soluble drugs have larger values which may, as seen above for nortriptyline, greatly exceed the physical volume available for distribution in the subject. For this reason the volume determined from experimental results is called the *apparent volume of distribution, V*.

5.3.1 *Partition coefficient*

If it is considered that the subject has a fixed physical volume of distribution, the varying values of V for different drugs may be expressed by means of a partition coefficient, P, for the distribution from plasma to outer volume for each drug.

A value of P much less than 1 means that, as with gentamicin and salicylate, the distribution is limited; values much larger than 1 indicate strong binding of the drug in the outer volume.

The apparent volume of distribution of a drug may be assessed from the total area under the C, t curve, as explained in Section 9.5.

6. ENZYME KINETICS AND DRUG METABOLISM

6.1 Enzyme kinetics

Enzymes act as catalysts for most *in vivo* chemical reactions. They are macromolecules and in the presence of an excess of the reacting substance (the substrate) the enzyme surface becomes saturated and the reaction proceeds at a constant rate, giving zero-order kinetics.

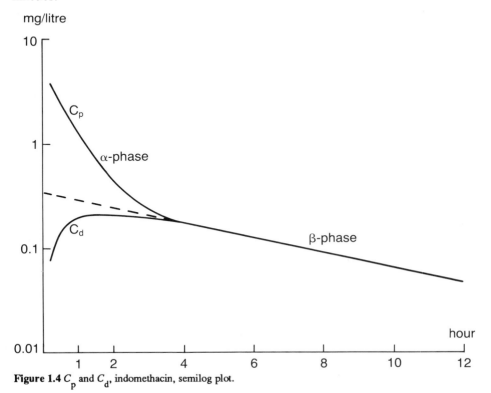

Figure 1.4 C_p and C_d, indomethacin, semilog plot.

As the substrate concentration falls, the degree of saturation declines and the rate becomes dependent on the substrate concentration. At low substrate concentrations, the rate becomes proportional to the concentration, giving first-order kinetics.

These results are summarized in the Michaelis–Menten equation for enzyme kinetics, as with the zero-order equation the rate, rate(X), is expressed as rate of change of amount X of drug, with time.

$$\text{rate}(X) = -V_{max} \times C_s/(K_m + C_s)$$

(1.3)

The sign is negative because X decreases as time increases. Rate(X) is the rate of change of amount of substrate in mg/h; V_{max} is the maximum rate at saturation, in mg/h; C_s is the substrate concentration in mg/l; K_m is the Michaelis constant in mg/l.

By substituting $C_s = K_m$ into this equation we get

$$\text{rate}(X) = -V_{max}/2$$

and so K_m may be thought of as the concentration at which the rate of reaction is half the maximum rate.

At high concentrations with C_s considerably greater than K_m, $C_s/(K_m + C_s)$ becomes approximately equal to 1 and rate(X) becomes equal to $-V_{max}$ giving zero-order kinetics.

At low concentrations $C_s/(K_m + C_s)$ becomes approximately C_s/K_m and the rate becomes

$$\text{rate}(X) = -(V_{max}/K_m)C_s$$

which is a first-order kinetic equation with rate proportional to concentration. These effects are shown in *Figures 1.5* and *1.6*.

Figure 1.5 is an X, t plot of data calculated from the Michaelis–Menten equation:

$$\text{rate}(X) = -20 \times C/(10 + C) \text{ mg/h}$$

The initial part of the plot, where the rate is equal to $-V_{max}$, is linear, later it becomes curved as the Michaelis–Menten equation takes over.

Figure 1.6 shows the same data plotted on semilog paper. The initial curved part of the graph is the region of zero order and Michaelis–Menten kinetics, the final linear part of the graph is the first-order region.

6.2 Drug metabolism kinetics

Drugs are mainly metabolized by enzymes in the liver. Therapeutic concentrations are usually low enough for the metabolic reactions to be first-order. However, some important drugs such as phenytoin and aspirin show enzyme saturation (capacity-limited effect) in the therapeutic range of plasma concentration. The medical consequence of this type of kinetics is that an increase in dose produces a disproportionate increase in plasma concentration, which may lead to toxicity. This situation is discussed more fully in Chapter 7.

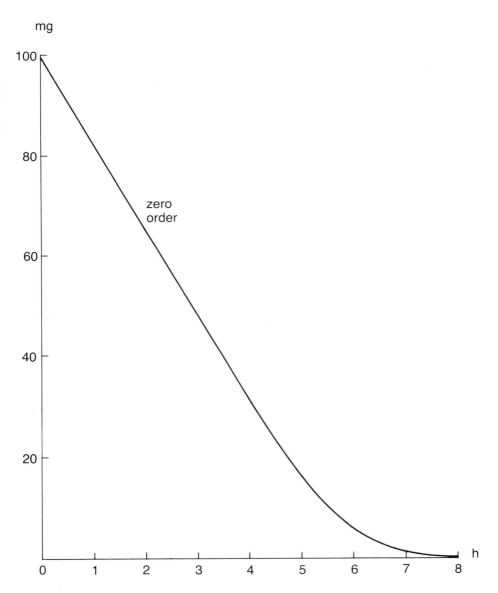

Figure 1.5 Capacity-limited kinetics, X, t plot.

With a drug showing capacity-limited kinetics, it is the relative values of the therapeutic plasma concentration and the parameter K_m of the Michaelis–Menten equation which determine how significant the effect is likely to be.

For example, paracetamol has K_m around 30 mg/l and a minimum active plasma level C_{act} of around 5 mg/l. The capacity-limited effect is therefore of little significance in the therapeutic range of doses; however, it is important in cases where an overdose has been taken (Chapter 8, Sections 3–5).

With phenytoin, K_m is around 7 mg/l and C_{act} around 10 mg/l; therapeutic doses will therefore produce significant enzyme-saturation effects.

For capacity-limited drug metabolism, V_{max} is usually expressed in amount of drug per unit time, e.g. mg/h.

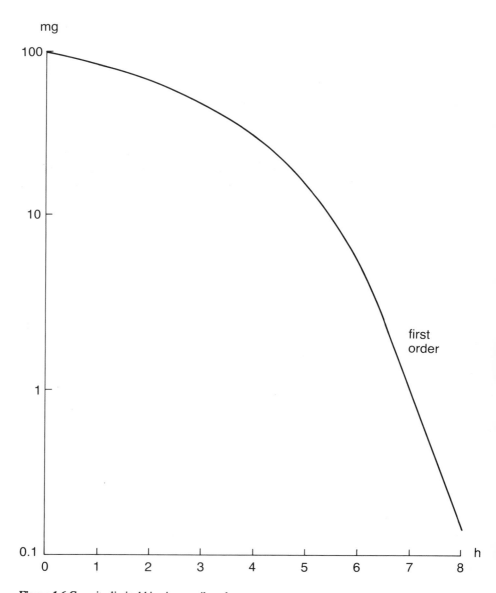

Figure 1.6 Capacity-limited kinetics, semilog plot.

6.3 Types of drug metabolism

Most primary metabolic reactions involve oxidation of the drug to more polar substances which are then more readily excreted in the urine. In addition, drug and primary metabolite molecules may be conjugated, i.e. chemically attached, to polar entities such as glucuronide, uric acid or sulphate; this conjugation additionally facilitates excretion. The more polar drug metabolites are mostly inactive and are rapidly eliminated.

Other than oxidation, hydrolysis, demethylation and reduction may also occur.

6.3.1 *Pro-drugs*

A pro-drug is an inactive substance which is more readily absorbed than the active drug or which avoids adverse effects caused by oral dosing with the active drug. The pro-drug is converted to the active form, after absorption, by *in vivo* metabolism.

For example, esters of ampicillin such as pivampicillin and talampicillin are more completely absorbed after an oral dose than ampicillin itself. After absorption they are rapidly hydrolysed to ampicillin. Use of the esters also reduces the incidence of diarrhoea.

Although the liver is the principal site for metabolic reactions, they may also occur at other sites; enzymes in the blood, the kidney, the gastro-intestinal tract (GIT) and the lung may play a part in the metabolism of some drugs.

6.4 Hepatic mechanisms

The liver receives about 30% of the cardiac output of blood, in two supplies. The first is from the hepatic artery and the second is from the hepatic portal vein, which carries blood from the vessels perfusing the stomach and intestine. This second supply contains substances, including drugs, which have been absorbed from the GIT.

The arterial blood is oxygenated and so when the two supplies mix together in the region of the liver cells, conditions favourable for the oxidation of the absorbed molecules are established.

Molecules of unchanged drug and its metabolite pass on from the liver cells to the hepatic vein where they join the general blood circulation.

A flow of bile, a solubilizing fluid, is produced in the liver and passes on to the gall bladder and then to the intestine. Most drugs and their metabolites dissolve to some extent in the bile and are transported from the liver to the lower intestine. They are then either excreted in the faeces or reabsorbed back into the plasma.

The bile flow is slow, around 0.6 ml/min; biliary excretion of a drug is therefore small unless, like ampicillin, the drug concentrates in the bile.

These hepatic processes are shown diagrammatically in *Figure 1.7*.

6.5 First-pass metabolism (pre-systemic metabolism)

A drug given by the oral route is absorbed from the GIT into the portal blood circulation, which carries it directly to the liver before any outer distribution occurs. Consequently in the first pass through the liver the drug is at a much higher concentration than it is after distribution has taken place.

This situation may produce a substantial metabolism of the drug before it reaches the main plasma volume, giving rise to the *first-pass effect*.

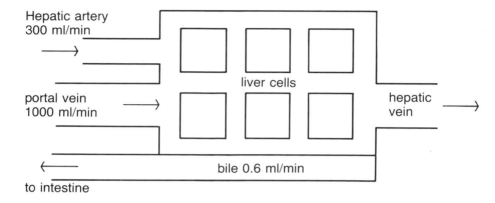

Figure 1.7 Diagram for liver function.

The fraction of the amount of drug taken up into the plasma from an oral dose, which is metabolized in the first-pass effect is called the *liver extraction ratio, E*. With some drugs it has a high value, making the oral route an inefficient method for administering the drug.

Nortriptyline has a value of E of about 0.5, meaning that half of an oral dose is metabolized before it reaches the main plasma volume; however, the metabolites formed are not toxic and so the oral route is used. Lignocaine has a value of E of 0.65, and one of the metabolites formed is more toxic than the parent drug: the oral route is therefore not used with this drug.

6.6 Enzyme induction

Some drugs have the ability to induce the production of hepatic enzymes. This enzyme induction may manifest itself as an increase in the clearance of the inducing drug as well as of certain other drugs which may be co-prescribed. During chronic dosing, enzyme induction may cause plasma concentrations to fall to sub-optimal levels.

Examples are rifampicin, phenobarbitone and carbamazepine. The latter two are anticonvulsants used in long-term treatment. Rifampicin, an antituberculous agent, is capable of increasing the clearance of theophylline by 25%. The induction effect is slow to develop, but after several weeks the mean plasma concentration may decline from an initially active level to an inactive one.

The consequences of enzyme induction are discussed in Chapter 5, Section 6.3.

6.7 Enzyme inhibition

Inhibition of hepatic enzyme activity may be produced by a number of drugs such as cimetidine, isoniazid and erythromycin. Unlike enzyme induction, which is slow to develop, enzyme inhibition normally ocurs as soon as the inhibiting drug is added to a patient's treatment, although it may take several days in some cases to reach its peak effect. Examples of this sort of drug interaction include the inhibition of theophylline metabolism by ciprofloxacin (a new quinolone antibiotic), cimetidine and erythromycin and the inhibition of both warfarin and phenytoin metabolism by cimetidine.

The effect of ciprofloxacin on theophylline clearance is the most dramatic and figures as high as 65% reduction in clearance may be seen [A.H.Thomson, G.D.Thomson, M.Hepburn and B.Whiting, *Eur. J. Clin. Pharmacol.*, (1987) **33**, 435–436]. As a result of this, theophylline toxicity is frequently seen if appropriate dosage reduction and therapeutic drug monitoring are not effected.

7. DRUG ELIMINATION

7.1 Routes of elimination

The main route for the elimination of most drugs is urinary excretion of the unchanged drug and of its metabolites. For some drugs given by the oral route, there is incomplete absorption from the GIT and a substantial part of the dose is excreted in the faeces; an example is ampicillin.

Other routes of elimination are through the bile, leading to faecal excretion, through the skin and via the lungs. These are usually minor routes.

Urinary analyses following a drug dose provide a method for studying the extent of metabolism of a drug and for identifying the metabolites.

7.2 Renal mechanisms

About one-quarter of the cardiac output goes to the kidneys. Partial filtration occurs in the glomeruli and the filtrate contains only relatively small molecules, the plasma proteins and substances bound to them are retained in the blood. The filtrate passes on through the kidney tubules where it is in contact with a capillary network, through which the blood from the glomeruli flows.

In the tubules, most of the water from the filtrate is reabsorbed into the capillary blood as are less polar, small molecules. More polar molecules remain in the filtrate and pass on to be excreted in the urine.

Some highly polar molecules, such as the penicillins, undergo a secretion process in the tubules, whereby additional drug is transferred from the blood in the capillaries to the filtrate. Such drugs are very rapidly excreted in the urine.

These renal processes are shown diagrammatically in *Figure 1.8*. The rates of flow shown are estimates for a 70-kg male. The 1400 ml/min blood flow to the kidney provides 125 ml/min of glomerular filtrate; after tubular reabsorption of water, this flow is reduced to 1 ml/min of urine formation.

The concentration of unbound drug in the glomerular filtrate is equal to that in the plasma, $(1 - F_b)C$, and the rate of removal of the drug into the filtrate in mg/h is equal to this concentration multiplied by the glomerular filtration rate, *GFR* in l/h. If there is no tubular reabsorption or secretion, the rate of urinary excretion of the drug, rate$(X)_u$ (in mg/h), is then equal to this rate of removal.

$$\text{rate}(X)_u = GFR \times (1 - F_b)C$$

rate$(X)_u$ is the rate of elimination in mg/h; *GFR* is the glomerular fitration rate in l/h; F_b

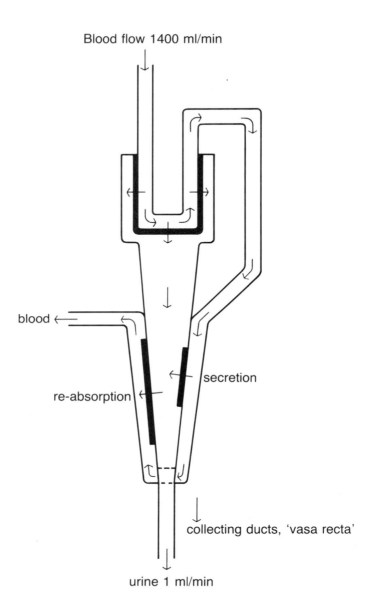

Blood flow 1400 ml/min

blood ←

re-absorption

secretion

collecting ducts, 'vasa recta'

urine 1 ml/min

Figure 1.8 Diagram for kidney function. (Thick lines indicate regions where transfer occurs.)

is the fraction of the drug in the plasma which is bound to protein; C is the plasma concentration.

The effects of reabsorption and secretion of the drug in the tubules may be accounted for by means of a dimensionless renal tubular function RTF, which is introduced as a dividing factor into the equation for rate$(X)_u$.

$$\text{rate}(X)_u = GFR \times (1 - F_b)C/RTF$$

(1.4)

If the drug is not reabsorbed or secreted in the tubules, $RTF = 1$; when there is net re-absorption into the blood in the tubules, as occurs with less polar drugs, RTF is greater than 1; when there is net secretion in the tubules, as with the penicillins, RTF is less than 1.

8. THE UPTAKE AND DISPOSITION OF A DRUG

The disposition of a drug includes distribution, metabolism, excretion and all the processes which the drug undergoes after uptake.The uptake of a drug into the plasma depends on the route of administration. With the i.v. route the drug is injected directly into the blood; with the oral route, the uptake is by absorption of drug from the GIT; with the intramuscular (i.m.) and other routes, uptake is by absorption from a parenteral depot.

Figure 1.9 illustrates the uptake and disposition processes.

8.1 Intravenous route of administration

When a drug is given by the i.v. route all the dose enters the plasma. An i.v. bolus is a rapid injection of the drug which then becomes completely mixed throughout the plasma in about 1 min. For an i.v. infusion, a solution containing the drug is slowly infused into the blood at a uniform rate.

As soon as the drug enters the plasma, protein binding and distribution to the outer volume commence; when it reaches the liver, metabolism starts and there is some dissolution of drug in the bile; when the drug and its metabolites reach the kidneys, excretion in the urine begins.

8.2 Oral route of administration

Drug given by the oral route passes into the stomach and then into the intestine. There is some absorption from the stomach but the main absorption into the plasma is in the small intestine. The absorbed drug passes into the portal circulation and the drug is carried directly to the liver before any distribution can occur, giving rise to the first-pass effect described in Section 6.5.

The shape of a typical C, t plot following an oral dose is shown in *Figure 1.10*. After an initial lag time before a measurable amount of drug appears in the plasma, C rises as the drug is absorbed, to a maximum at which the rate of absorption and the sum of the rates of distribution and elimination become balanced; C subsequently declines.

8.2.1 *Lag time*

When the oral dosage form is a tablet or capsule, there may be a significant time before the dosage form releases sufficient drug for it to be detectable in the plasma. This time after dose during which the plasma concentration is zero is called the lag time.

21

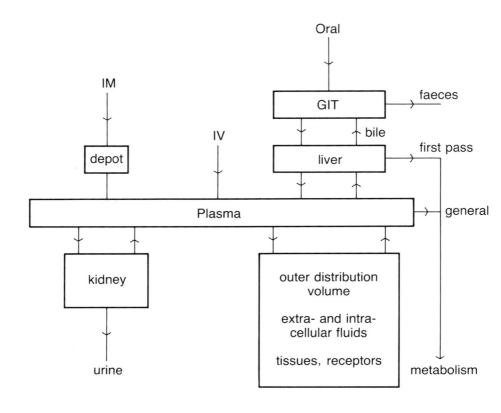

Figure 1.9 Uptake and disposition in the simulation model.

Lag time may be estimated by determining C at short intervals after dose and extrapolating the C, t plot to zero C. The lag time is then the intercept on the time axis, as shown in *Figure 1.10*.

When an oral dose is given as a solution or suspension, the lag time is often negligible.

8.2.2 *Absorption*

Absorption from the GIT may be considered to be a first-order process with the rate proportional to the amount of drug available for absorption, which remains in the GIT. Absorption is often incomplete with the unabsorbed drug passing to excretion in the faeces.

The fraction of an oral dose D, which is absorbed from the GIT into the plasma is denoted by F_a. The fraction unabsorbed $(1 - F_a)$ also includes drug which is transported from the liver via the bile to excretion in the faeces, since this amount does not enter the general blood circulation.

The value of F_a may sometimes be determined experimentally by analysing urine samples for the parent drug and its metabolites, over a period long enough for complete excretion of an oral dose of the drug. The estimation of F_a in the simplified situation of the computer model is straightforward; however, in reality there are often many complicating factors.

8.2.3 *Bioavailability*

The fraction F, of an oral dose which reaches the plasma intact is called the bioavailability. F is normally less than 1, due to incomplete absorption and the first-pass effect.

Bioavailability may be determined from experimental measurements of areas under C, t plots (Section 9.4).

8.2.4 *Late time plasma half-life*

At later times following an oral dose, the $\log(C)$, t plot becomes linear. When the elimination rate constant is less than the absorption rate constant, which is often the case, the slope of this plot gives the same plasma half-life as that found following an i.v. dose, equal to $0.693/k$. However, if the two rate constants are similar, the plasma half-life is affected by the continuing absorption and is longer than that found by analysis of i.v. route data.

8.2.5 *Liver extraction ratio*

The amount of an oral dose D taken up from a dosage form is $F_a \times D$ and the amount metabolized in the first pass is $F_a \times D \times E$, where E is the liver extraction ratio. The amount absorbed which is not metabolized is therefore $F_a \times D(1 - E)$. The fraction of the dose reaching the plasma intact is $F_a(1 - E)$ and this is the bioavailability F.

Thus we have:

$$F = F_a(1 - E)$$

and by rearranging:

$$E = 1 - F/F_a$$

(1.5)

This equation may be used to estimate the liver extraction ratio from values of F and F_a.

8.2.6 *Sustained release*

When a sustained release preparation is used for oral dosage, the rate of absorption may be better expressed as two consecutive constant rate (zero-order) processes (Chapter 6, Section 2).

8.3 Intramuscular and other routes

Drug given by the i.m. route forms a depot in the muscle from which it is absorbed into the plasma. The absorption may be described as a first-order process.

There is no first-pass effect since the drug goes directly into the main blood circulation. There may be a lag time and though with most drugs uptake is complete, there are exceptions.

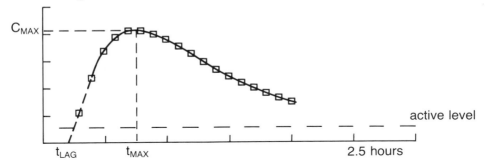

C,t plot indomethacin 25 mg PO
Subject, 25 y, 70 kg, 183 cm, male
2500 microg/litre

Figure 1.10 Oral dose C, t plot; 25 mg indomethacin.

An example of a drug exhibiting incomplete uptake from an i.m. depot is phenytoin. Plasma concentrations following i.m. injection are only about half those with the same dose given orally. This effect is thought to be due to precipitation of phenytoin at the site of injection [A.Richens, *Clin. Pharmacokin.*,(1979), **4**, 153–169]. Another example is ampicillin; the results of T.Bergan [*Antimicrob. Agents Chemother.*,(1978), **13**, 971–974] on plasma concentrations following equal i.v. and i.m. doses indicate that uptake from the i.m. dose is incomplete.

Other cases of apparent incomplete uptake from an i.m. dose may be due to prolonged slow absorption, giving rise to plasma levels below the limit of detection of the drug.

As $E = 0$, then $F = F_a$ for the i.m. route; the bioavailability is equal to the fraction of the dose which is taken up into the plasma.

Other routes of administration include transdermal, sublingual and rectal administration of drug. As with the i.m. route, a depot of drug is set up, from which it is absorbed into the general blood circulation, avoiding presystemic metabolism.

8.4 Combined rate equation

The processes of uptake and disposition may be quantified and combined to give an equation for the rate of change of plasma concentration of drug with time.

$$\text{rate}(C) = \text{rate}(C)_{uptk} - \text{rate}(C)_d - \text{rate}(C)_m - \text{rate}(C)_u$$

where: $\text{rate}(C)$ = total rate of change of plasma concentration; the other rates are components of the total, contributed by the processes indicated by the subscripts: uptk for uptake, d for outward distribution, m for metabolism and u for urinary excretion.

The rates all need to be expressed in terms of change of plasma concentration per unit time, mg/(l h).

The rate of uptake is dose and route dependent and will consist of zero-order terms for i.v. infusion and for oral sustained release; for ordinary oral doses and for i.m. injection, it will consist of a first-order term.

24

The rate of distribution describes the rate of transfer of drug from plasma to the outer distribution volume. This transfer is taken as first order; the rate constant acts on the difference between the plasma concentration of the drug and the mean concentration in the outer apparent distribution volume. The flow ceases when the two concentrations become equal and they subsequently decline together.

The rate of metabolism of the drug may follow first-order or capacity-limited kinetics. The rate of urinary excretion is normally first-order, the rate constant applying to the plasma concentration.

Combined rate equations are complicated; if all the rates are first-order they can be solved to give C at defined times and these results can be compared with experimental values so as to evaluate the rate constants involved.

A more detailed discussion of combined rate equations is given in Appendix I, Section 5.

9. AREA UNDER THE PLASMA CONCENTRATION–TIME CURVE

9.1 Area determination

Experimental C, t values are subject to scatter due to unavoidable experimental error in the determination of C. One of the most reliable quantities which can be estimated from such scattered data is the area under the curve, since all the points are used and the scatter tends to average out.

The area under an experimental C, t plot is approximately determined by dividing it into vertical strips at each experimental point as shown in *Figure 1.11*. The tops of the strips are taken as straight lines and so each strip forms a trapezium of area equal to base × mean height. The strip areas are calculated from the data values and added together to give an estimate of the area under the curve.

As an example, the data plotted in *Figure 1.11* are:

t (h)	C (mg/l)	t (h)	C (mg/l)
0.25	14.3	2.0	7.80
0.5	14.3	3.0	5.74
0.75	12.7	4.0	4.36
1.0	11.4	6.0	2.58
1.25	10.2	8.0	1.54
1.5	9.30		

Initially, while the concentration values are changing rapidly, results are taken at short intervals, the intervals are opened out later. The strip (trapezium) areas are:

strip 1 $0.25 \times (0 + 14.3)/2$ =   1.79
strip 2 $0.25 \times (14.3 + 14.3)/2$ =   3.58
strip 3 $0.25 \times (14.3 + 12.7)/2$ =   3.38

strip 4 $0.25 \times (12.7 + 11.4)/2$	=	3.01
strip 5 $0.25 \times (11.4 + 10.2)/2$	=	2.70
strip 6 $0.25 \times (10.2 + 9.3)/2$	=	2.44
strip 7 $0.5 \times (9.3 + 7.8)/2$	=	4.28
strip 8 $1.0 \times (7.8 + 5.74)/2$	=	6.77
strip 9 $1.0 \times (5.74 + 4.36)/2$	=	5.05
strip 10 $2.0 \times (4.36 + 2.58)/2$	=	6.94
strip 11 $2.0 \times (2.58 + 1.54)/2$	=	4.12

sum   44.1 h mg/l

The first trapezium is in fact a triangle (one vertical side equal to zero).

If the experiment had been continued for a longer period, a further contribution to the total area would have been obtained.

The design of an experiment to obtain a reliable estimate of the area under a C, t plot is discussed in detail in Chapter 2, Section 4.2. Calculations of area are tedious and a computer program to carry them out is very helpful.

9.2 Total area

An experiment to determine total area should be continued until the plasma concentration has become negligible; however, this may mean a very long experiment. An alternative method is to make a run for about three half-lives, estimate this area by the trapezium rule and add on an extrapolation term to estimate the total area to infinite time.

If the area up to time t_n is denoted by area$_n$, the extrapolation term by area$_e$, the total area by area$_T$ and the plasma concentration at time t_n by C_n, then the extrapolation term is (Appendix I, Section 2.2):

$$\text{area}_e = C_n/k$$

where k is the late-time, first-order elimination constant for the drug.

The total area is therefore:

$$\text{area}_T = \text{area}_n + C_n/k$$

(1.6)

In the example shown in *Figure 1.11*, the late-time elimination constant is estimated as $0.26\,\text{h}^{-1}$; C_n, the last concentration, is 1.54 mg/l, therefore the extrapolation term is $1.54/0.26 = 5.9$ h mg/l, giving a total area:

$$\text{area}_T = 44.1 + 5.9 = 50.0 \text{ h mg/l}$$

9.3 Theoretical significance of area

Each strip area in the determination by the trapezium method is the mean plasma concentration of the drug over the strip time interval, multiplied by the time for which this mean concentration operates; the total area is consequently proportional to the amount of drug which has passed through the plasma; the theoretical significance of area is based

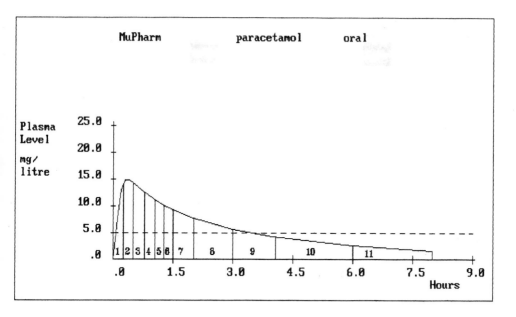

Figure 1.11 Area by the trapezium method; paracetamol 100 mg oral.

on this conclusion, which is discussed further in Section 9.4 and demonstrated in Appendix I, Section 2.1.

9.4 Area and bioavailability

The proportionality between area and amount of drug passing through the plasma is the basis for the use of area determinations to estimate bioavailability. For example, to find the bioavailability of a drug given by the oral route, a dose D mg is administered to a subject and plasma concentrations are determined at suitable intervals for estimating area. The study is then repeated *with the same subject or group of subjects*, and with the same or lower dose given as an i.v. infusion over a period of about 0.5 h (i.v. bolus dose leads to high, rapidly changing C values) and the i.v. area is determined.

By the i.v. route the whole dose enters directly into the plasma; by the oral route only $F \times D$ mg of drug reaches the plasma intact. The ratio of the two areas measures the ratio of the amounts of drug passing through the plasma as a result of dosing by the two routes, and so the ratio of areas provides an estimate of the bioavailability from the oral route.

$$F = \text{area}_T(D \text{ mg, oral})/\text{area}_T(D \text{ mg, i.v. infusion})$$

$$(1.7)$$

An experiment to estimate bioavailability from an oral dose is described in Chapter 3, Section 2.

9.5 Area and volume of distribution

The mean value of C over the period of a run is equal to the area under the C,t curve divided by the length of the run (mean value theorem).

Consider a plasma concentration–time study with a single dose D mg of a drug, lasting for a time t h, sufficiently long for C to have declined to zero at time t. The area under the curve is then area$_T$ and the mean value of C over the whole period is:

$$C_{mean} = \text{area}_T/t \text{ mg/l}$$

(1.8)

If the elimination is first order and k h^{-1} is the first-order rate constant, the rate of elimination at any time is rate of elimination $= k \times C$ mg/(1 h). To convert the rate to mg/h, this expression is multipled by the total volume in which the drug is distributed, V1: rate of elimination in mg/h$= V \times k \times C$. The mean rate of elimination over the whole period is rate $(X)_e = V \times k \times C_{mean}$ mg/h. If this mean rate is multiplied by the duration of the experiment, t h, we get the total amount of drug eliminated: total eliminated$= V \times k \times C_{mean} \times t$ mg. Substituting for C_{mean}, the t values cancel, leaving total eliminated $= V \times k \times \text{area}_T$ mg.

The total eliminated is equal to the total amount of drug which has passed through the plasma, $F \times D$, where F is the bioavailability by the route of administration used:

$$F \times D = V \times k \times \text{area}_T$$

(1.9)

This equation has many applications in pharmacokinetics, an alternative derivation in terms of calculus is given in Appendix I, Section 3. Its use for assessing the mean apparent volume of distribution is exemplified in Chapter 2, Section 4.3.

9.6 Other applications of area estimates

The use of area for calculating the total clearance of a drug is described in Section 10.3 and Chapter 2, Section 4.3.

The total clearance may then be used for designing repeated dosing schedules for a drug from single-dose results (Chapter 5, Section 3).

Area values at different doses of a drug may be used for detecting capacity-limited kinetics in the disposition of a drug (Chapter 7, Section 3).

10. CLEARANCE

10.1 General definition of clearance

The concept of clearance is an important one in the application of pharmacokinetics to medicine.

Consider an amount of drug X mg, at a concentration of C mg/l in a total volume (plasma

+ outer volume) of V litre, which is passed via the plasma through an eliminating organ. If ΔX is the amount eliminated in time Δt:

$$\text{rate of elimination} = \Delta X/\Delta t \ \text{mg/h}$$

ΔX mg occupies a volume $\Delta X/C$ l and this is the volume which is cleared completely of drug in time Δt.

$$\text{rate of clearance} = (\Delta X/C)/\Delta t \ \text{l/h}$$

The term *clearance*, Cl, is defined as this rate. Rearranging the above equation:

$$Cl = (\Delta X/\Delta t)/C$$

(1.10)

or   clearance = (rate of elimination, mg/h)/(plasma concentration, mg/l) l/h

The above equation gives a practical definition of clearance. It is seen that clearance multiplied by plasma concentration gives a convenient estimate of the rate of elimination of a drug by a particular route.

An important property of clearance is that when the elimination process is first-order, the clearance is constant for a given subject and independent of C (Appendix I, Section 4.2). When the elimination is capacity limited, the clearance decreases as the value of C increases (Chapter 7, Section 3.3).

10.2 Renal clearance

Renal elimination is generally first-order. It may be determined accurately in a subject by giving the drug as an i.v. infusion. When a constant plasma concentration has been attained a urine sample is collected to assess the rate of urinary excretion. The above equation (1.10) is then used to calculate Cl_r, the renal clearance.

This procedure involves a special experiment; it is usually more convenient to calculate renal clearance from urine and plasma concentrations of a drug during a course of treatment.

If the drug is given by the oral route the values of C will be varying. Plasma samples are taken at two suitable times after dose, the first at t_1 should be after a long enough period for most of the absorption to be complete, the second at t_2 should be such that C has not changed too much but a measurable amount of drug has been eliminated in the urine.

A urine sample is collected over the interval t_1 to t_2 and analysed to determine the amount of drug excreted in the urine, ΔX_u, over this period. The mean rate of excretion over the interval is then $\Delta X_u/(t_2 - t_1)$ mg/h.

If C_1 and C_2 are the plasma concentrations in mg/l, the mean concentration over the interval is $C_{mean} = (C_1 + C_2)/2$.

To estimate Cl_r, the mean excretion rate is divided by the mean plasma concentration giving a final equation for Cl_r:

$$Cl_r = [\Delta X_u/(t_2 - t_1)]/C_{mean}$$

(1.11)

29

To illustrate the use of this equation the following data were obtained after a 250 mg i.v. bolus dose of kanamycin: $t_1 = 3$ h; $C_1 = 9.2$ mg/l; $t_2 = 4$ h; $C_2 = 6.6$ mg/l; ΔX_u = amount excreted in the urine between 3 and 4 h = 41.1 mg; the mean rate of excretion, rate$(X)_u$, is therefore 41.1 mg/h; $C_{mean} = (9.2 + 6.6)/2 = 7.9$ mg/l.

Using the formula $Cl_r = \text{rate}(X)_u/C_{mean}$:

$$Cl_r = 41.1/7.9 = 5.2 \text{ l/h}$$

This value is somewhat below GFR, which for this subject is 7.1 l/h.

A more accurate method is to determine C at one or more times between t_1 and t_2; the area under the C,t curve between t_1 and t_2, area$_{12}$, is estimated by the trapezium rule. Then since

$$C_{mean} = \text{area}_{12}/(t_2 - t_1)$$

equation (1.11) becomes

$$Cl_r = \Delta X_u/\text{area}_{12}$$

10.3 Total clearance

Renal clearance of a drug may be readily determined from experimental studies. The total clearance of a drug is calculated from a definition similar to that for Cl_r.

Consider an experiment in which a dose D is given, of which a fraction F is taken up into the plasma, and plasma levels suitable for area calculation are determined at a series of times up to $t = T$ h, where T is sufficiently large for total elimination of the drug to have occurred.

The mean value of C over the whole time period is

$$C_{mean} = \text{area}_T/T$$

The total elimination over the period T is $F \times D$ mg, giving a mean rate of elimination of $(F \times D)/T$ mg/h.

The total clearance Cl_T is then defined as

$$Cl_T = \text{mean rate of elimination/mean plasma concentration}$$

or

$$Cl_T = (F \times D/T)/(\text{area}_T/T)$$

The two T values cancel giving

$$Cl_T = F \times D/\text{area}_T$$

(1.12)

10.4 Hepatic clearance

Hepatic clearance Cl_h may be defined in the same way as renal clearance but it is not readily measurable experimentally. It is usually assessed as the difference between Cl_T and Cl_r:

$$Cl_h = Cl_T - Cl_r$$

(1.13)

An example of the calculations of all three clearances is given in Chapter 2, Section 4.3.

10.5 Renal clearance and experimental measurement of glomerular filtration rate

In Section 7.2 it was seen that the rate of urinary elimination in mg/h is given by

$$\text{rate}(X)_u = GFR \times (1 - F_b) \times C/RTF$$

If a substance is not bound to plasma protein ($F_b = 0$) and is neither reabsorbed nor secreted in the tubules ($RTF = 1$):

$$\text{rate}(X)_u = GFR \times C \quad \text{or} \quad GFR = \text{rate}(X)_u/C$$

The renal clearance is (rate of elimination)/C:

$$Cl_r = \text{rate}(X)_u/C = GFR$$

Estimation of the renal clearance of such a substance therefore gives a method of measuring the *glomerular filtration rate* of the subject.

GFR depends on the characteristics of a subject. For a 70-kg, 25-year-old male an average value is 7.5 l/h or 125 ml/min.

10.5.1 *Inulin*

A substance which has the properties required for measuring GFR is inulin, a plant polysaccharide of molecular mass around 5000. In addition to these requirements, it is not metabolized *in vivo* and so all the clearance is through the kidneys.

For determining GFR, the subject is given an i.v. bolus dose of inulin of 3 mg followed by an i.v.infusion of 7 mg/h. With the 25-year-old male, a steady plasma level of 0.93 mg/l is rapidly attained. A urine sample from 2 to 3 h after dose shows that 7.01 mg is excreted in this period.

The rate of excretion is therefore 7.01 mg/h, while the value of C is constant at 0.93 mg/l. The renal clearance is therefore

$$Cl_r = 7.01/0.93 = 7.54 \text{ l/h} = 126 \text{ ml/min}$$

and Cl_r is the value of GFR for this subject.

10.5.2 *Creatinine*

Another substance with suitable properties for GFR determination is creatinine. This substance is produced in the body at a constant rate for a given subject, it is present in the serum (plasma) at a steady-state concentration C_{cr} mg/l, at which the rate of formation rate $(X_{cr})_{form}$ mg/h is equal to the rate of elimination. The latter is equal to clearance times plasma concentration. If X_{cr} is the amount of creatinine,

$$\text{rate}(X_{cr})_{form} = Cl_r \times C_{cr} = GFR \times C_{cr}$$

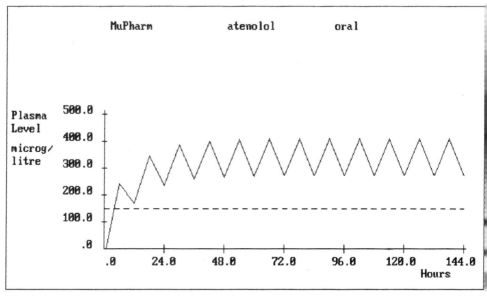

Press any key to continue

Figure 1.12 Atenolol 50 mg every 12 h, oral.

Since rate$(X_{cr})_{form}$ remains constant, determination of the serum (plasma) level of creatinine provides a method for monitoring whether any change has occurred in the *GFR* of a subject (see Chapter 8, Section 6.3 and Chapter 9, Section 6.1).

GFR provides an index of the renal function of a subject. When there is renal impairment, *GFR* decreases causing an increase in the serum concentration of creatinine.

11. REGIMENS WITH REPEATED DOSES. STEADY STATE

When a drug is given at intervals smaller than the time for complete elimination, the mean plasma concentration over each interval increases with each dose. For first-order elimination, the rate is proportional to plasma concentration and so the amount eliminated per unit time also increases, until the amount eliminated over a dosing interval becomes equal to the uptake of drug from each dose. At this point a steady state is reached at which the mean plasma concentration over each dosing interval becomes constant.

At the steady state, the plasma concentration varies during the dosing interval and these variations are exactly repeated over successive intervals. This effect is shown in *Figure 1.12* which shows plasma concentrations following oral doses of 50 mg of atenolol given every 12 h.

To be able to set up a multiple-dose regimen in which the drug is maintained above the minimum active plasma concentration and below the minimum toxic level, we need to be able to calculate the dose D, required at a given interval I_D, to produce a mean steady-state plasma concentration C_{SS}, which is between these two levels.

The length of the dosing interval I_D, is decided primarily on the basis of the half-life of the drug. With a drug of short half-life, a short interval is required to avoid too large a difference between peak and trough plasma concentrations within the interval. With drugs of long half-life, a 24-h interval is usually used. Further consideration of the dosing interval is given in Chapter 5, Section 3.3.

The calculation of dose may be made for drugs having first-order disposition kinetics, by considering the total clearance Cl_T.

From the definition of Cl_T:

$$\text{rate}(X)_e = Cl_T \times C$$

where $\text{rate}(X)_e$ is the rate of elimination of a drug in mg/h and C is the plasma concentration in mg/l.

The amount eliminated over the dosing interval I_D is

$$X_e = I_D \times \text{rate}(X)_e = I_D \times Cl_T \times C_{\text{mean}}$$

where C_{mean} is the mean value of C over the interval.

At the steady state, C_{mean} becomes C_{SS}, the mean steady-state plasma concentration over the dosing interval, and the amount eliminated becomes equal to $F \times D$, the amount of drug taken up from the dose, where F is the bioavailability. The condition for the steady state is therefore

$$F \times D = I_D \times Cl_T \times C_{SS}$$

F and Cl_T may be determined experimentally from area runs; C_{SS} is given a suitable target value; I_D is fixed in relation to the half-life of the drug and to clinical factors. From these values, the required value of D given at intervals I_D may be assessed.

$$D = I_D \times Cl_T \times C_{SS}/F$$

$$(1.14)$$

The need for an i.v. run to determine bioavailability may be avoided by making a run for area with a single dose D_1 given by the route being used, e.g. the oral route.

By equation (1.12):

$$Cl_T = F \times D_1/\text{area}_T(D_1,\text{oral})$$

Substituting this value of Cl_T in equation (1.14), F cancels since both D and D_1 are given by the same route and so are subject to the same bioavailability:

$$D = I_D \times C_{SS} \times D_1/\text{area}_T(D_1,\text{oral})$$

$$(1.15)$$

To use this equation to calculate the repeated dose, D, only one single dose run — to determine $\text{area}_T(D_1,\text{oral})$ — is required.

The use of these equations is further discussed, with experiments, in Chapters 5 and 6.

12. THE SIMULATION MODEL OF PHARMACOKINETICS

12.1 General description

The model of the uptake and disposition of a drug which is used in the subsequent chapters to carry out simulated experiments in drug kinetics with human subjects has been set up by developing expressions for the rates of uptake, distribution, metabolism and excretion of the drug. These rates are expressed in terms of the dose of drug, the route of administration and two sets of factors — one which characterizes the drug and the other which characterizes the subject.

A combination of the rates is used to express the rate of change of the amount of drug in the plasma.

Starting with appropriate values at the time of dose, time is increased by a small amount (the iteration time, 0.01 h) and from the rates obtained, the changes in amounts distributed, metabolized, excreted and present in the plasma are calculated. This process is repeated over as many iterations as are required for a run of length defined by the user.

The results may be printed out in numerical form, plotted as plasma concentration against time or displayed as a diagram showing the disposition of the drug, at times specified by the user.

12.2 Drug and subject factors

To give an initial overview of the scope of the model, the way in which the drug and subject factors are combined together is illustrated in *Figure 1.13* for the oral route: df( ) means the drug factor number shown in the bracket and similarly sf( ) means a numbered subject factor. The metabolism is assumed to be first-order. A fuller discussion of structure of the simulation model is given in Appendix V. Details of subject factors are in Appendix III and details of drug factors are in Appendix IV.

The oral dose D is given. It is multiplied by df(5), which is the fraction of the dose which is absorbed, and this amount enters the gastro-intestinal tract (GIT). The amount in this location at any time is X_{GI}.

The drug is absorbed from the GIT by a first-order process with a rate constant, the absorption constant, which is df(3). Absorbed drug is taken in the hepatic portal circulation directly into the liver.

The amount of drug in the liver is subjected to two processes: one is a first-order transfer to the main plasma volume governed by sf(2) which simulates the liver blood flow rate and is related to the cardiac output of the subject; the second process is the first-pass metabolism in the liver. In the simulation model, the amount metabolized is that, converted to inactive substances which go out of the circulation. The metabolic rate is controlled by df(10), the first-order rate constant, modified by sf(6), a measure of hepatic function.

sf(1) is the plasma volume, df(7) is the fraction bound to plasma proteins.

The intact drug from the liver, circulating in the plasma, is subjected to the three disposition processes: distribution, excretion and metabolism. The rate of distribution outside the plasma is governed by df(8); the apparent volume of distribution is controlled by sf(4), the physical outer volume of distribution of the subject, and df(9), the effective partition coefficient between outer volume and plasma.

Urinary excretion is controlled by sf(9), the glomerular filtration rate of the subject, and df(14), the renal tubular function for the drug.

Metabolism rate for the drug in the general circulation is governed by the same factors as those for the first-pass effect, df(10) and sf(6).

Various disease states in a subject may be simulated by altering the values of subject factors and, sometimes, drug factors. For example, reduction of sf(6) may be used to simulate hepatic dysfunction, and a reduction of sf(9) simulates renal dysfunction.

13. ACTIVE AND TOXIC PLASMA LEVELS FOR A DRUG

In the simulation model, the often complex relationship between plasma concentrations and a subject's responses to a drug has been simplified by defining minimum plasma levels for therapeutic activity C_{act}, for toxicity C_{tox} and for lethality C_{leth}.

These levels depend on the purpose for which the drug is given; a list of these uses may be obtained through the dialogue of the program (Chapter 2, Section 2).

With a number of drugs there are well-defined plasma concentrations for activity and toxicity, with others the levels are less certain; the relationship between activity and plasma concentration may also be more complex than can be fully represented by these fixed levels. In such cases the levels should be regarded as a means for defining targets for dosing regimens rather than as closely representing drug responses.

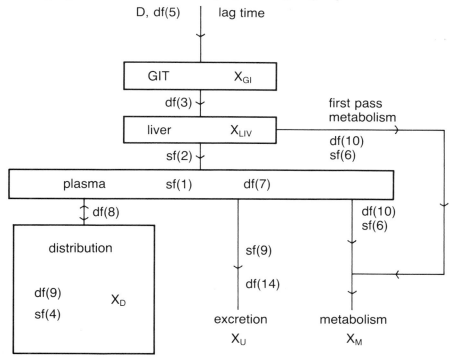

Figure 1.13 Oral dose, first-order metabolism.

Whatever the exact relationship between plasma concentration and response, the design of a multiple dosing schedule which will maintain a steady mean plasma concentration in an appropriate range between minimum activity and minimum toxicity is probably the best method for maintaining a continuous effective response to the drug.

Divergence between activity and plasma concentration occurs when the drug has a high affinity for the receptors responsible for the drug activity and when the receptors become saturated with drug. When the drug is strongly bound to the receptors the activity of the drug may decline more slowly than would be expected from the plasma concentrations — the drug activity persisting longer than would be expected from the plasma levels.

The importance of saturable effects (E_{max} type) in plasma concentration–response relationships has been discussed by Holford and Sheiner [H.G.H.Holford and L.B.Sheiner *Clin. Pharmacokin.*, (1981), 6, 429–453]. Saunders, Ingram and Warrington [L.Saunders, D.Ingram and S.J.Warrington J. *Pharm. Pharmacol.*, (1985), 37, 802–806] have studied data for exercise heart rate lowering resulting from administration of oxprenolol and have found that the plasma concentration-response is of this E_{max} type.

In the simulation, C_{act}, C_{tox} and C_{leth} are, wherever possible, based on values from the literature; the values used are listed in Appendix II.

A scheme of fixed levels of this type does not take into account the effects of inter-individual variation in the levels. However, all three levels are drug factors (Appendix IV) and may be readily changed by the user to give appropriate values for a particular subject. For example, if a subject is known to have developed tolerance to diamorphine, the three levels may be raised to appropriate values by changing the three drug factors in the dialogue of the simulation program.

CHAPTER 2

Single Intravenous Dose Experiments to Determine Pharmacokinetic Parameters. Studies with Gentamicin, Thiopentone, Ampicillin and Theophylline

1. PHARMACOKINETIC PARAMETERS

Some useful parameters for characterizing the pharmacokinetic behaviour of a drug following intravenous dose are: (i) plasma half-life; (ii) plasma elimination rate constant; (iii) area under the plasma-concentration – time curve; (iv) mean apparent volume of distribution; (v) renal clearance; and (vi) total clearance. These parameters have been defined in Chapter 1.

In addition, as discussed in Chapter 1, Section 5.2, the shape of the $\log(C),t$ curve following an i.v. bolus dose gives information about the time taken for a drug to penetrate the complete volume of distribution.

When an i.v. bolus dose is first given, the drug mixes rapidly in the plasma volume. As distribution proceeds outside the plasma, the effective volume occupied by the drug increases, reaching a maximum value. If this final volume is attained rapidly, as usually occurs with drugs of relatively small volumes of distribution, the plasma plus external volume occupied acts as a single unit and gives a straight line $\log(C),t$ plot (Chapter 1, Section 5.1 and Appendix I, Section 5.1). With drugs of high apparent volume of distribution, the time taken to reach the complete value is usually longer, resulting in a curved $\log(C),t$ plot.

2. SETTING UP A SIMULATED EXPERIMENT

Before setting up a simulated experiment in drug kinetics, as with a real one, the objectives need to be clearly defined and the experiment planned in detail.

Once the objectives have been defined and the dose and method of administration of the drug decided, then the times at which numerical results are required are selected, the subject is chosen and the dose is given.

In the simulation program the dialogue mirrors these stages clearly; questions are asked which require responses, and sets of alternative choices (menus) are presented. The user should have no difficulty in setting up an experiment which has been planned in advance. Full details of the dialogue are discussed in Chapter 4.

Table 2.1 Drugs in the simulation program and their uses. Active levels are set for the following uses of the drugs.

1.	Ampicillin, pneumonia	11.	Temazepam, sedation
2.	Aspirin, rheumatic fever	12.	Gentamicin, septicaemia
3.	Digitoxin, heart disease	13.	Digoxin, heart disease
4.	Indomethacin, pain relief	14.	Theophylline, asthma
5.	Kanamycin, septicaemia	15.	Lignocaine, arrhythmia
6.	Nortriptyline, depression	16.	Carbamazepine, convulsions
7.	Oxprenolol, hypertension	17.	Benzylpenicillin, meningitis
8.	Paracetamol, pain relief	18.	Thiopentone, anaesthetic
9.	Phenobarbitone, convulsions	19.	Atenolol, hypertension
10.	Phenytoin, convulsions	20.	Diamorphine, analgesic

The descriptions of the experiments are set out in this and subsequent chapters under the following headings: objectives, first plan, runs and results, second plan (if required), further runs and results (if required), conclusions.

At the end of each run, the program is reset for the same or for a different drug and at the end of the experiment, the program is stopped. If required, the results-log giving details of the full numerical results may then be printed out.

The first step in setting up a run is to load the computer program, named MuPharm, into the microcomputer. The details of this loading will depend on the machine used; information is given in the implementation notes supplied with the program.

On starting the program, introductory titles appear on the screen and remain until the <ENTER> key is pressed.

The dialogue commences with the DRUG SELECTION menu which shows the list of drugs available; by pressing 'q' or 'Q' (for query), followed by <ENTER>, the purposes for which the drugs are used in the simulation are shown as in *Table 2.1*.

3. EXPERIMENT 1: TO DETERMINE PHARMACOKINETIC PARAMETERS FOLLOWING INTRAVENOUS BOLUS DOSES OF GENTAMICIN AND THIOPENTONE

3.1 **Objectives**

This experiment is aimed at studying the shapes of the plasma concentration (C)–time (t) curves for the period soon after the injection is given, so as to illustrate differences in the times taken for the final volume of distribution to be penetrated.

Closely spaced results are required over a limited period; a run of 3 h with results every 0.1 h is suitable for both drugs.

3.2 **Plan of the experiment**

Half-lives and therapeutic doses for the drugs used in the simulation are listed in Appendix II, together with a summary of the drug properties. Gentamicin is an antibiotic and a suitable dose is 120 mg i.v. bolus; thiopentone is a short-acting anaesthetic, a suitable dose is 250 mg i.v. bolus. The timings for the results are every 0.1 h for 3 h — a total of 30 results for each run.

The subject used is the standard MuPharm subject, a 25-year-old male of body mass 70 kg and height 183 cm.

Options for the primary display of results are: a table of numerical values, a five-cycle semilog plot of C against t or a diagram showing the disposition of the drug. The chosen display appears as the calculations are made. At the end of the calculations, other types of presentation may be selected, the results having been stored in the computer memory for this pupose.

3.3 Runs and results

In the outline of the dialogue given below, the (sometimes abbreviated) requests and questions from the computer, the responses given by the user and the descriptions of the action are shown in a different typeface to the text; <E> indicates a press of the <ENTER> or the <RETURN> key.

3.3.1 *Gentamicin*

The dialogue starts with the choice of drug:

```
Enter number for drug        12 <E>     gentamicin
```

12 is the number shown in Table 2.1 for gentamicin.

On receiving the information for the choice of drug, the next screen display is the CONTROL menu which governs many of the subsequent operations. The 11 choices shown in Table 2.2 are discussed more fully in Chapter 4. Markers on the first three options indicate that these choices have to be made before a run can be started. As each of these choices is made, the marker for it disappears.

Table 2.2 The CONTROL menu.

```
CONTROL
         1. Prescribe Drug                <--
         2. Set timings for run           <--
         3. Specify subject               <--
         4. Change factors
         5. Start run at zero time
         6. Continue run
         7. Display results
         8. Estimate area under C,t plot
         9. Restart, same drug
        10. Restart, different drug
        11. Stop
```

The first option, `Prescribe drug`, is chosen; this leads to queries about details of the dose and the method of administration. The questions following are:

```
Enter dose in mg                 120 <E>

Multiple doses                   <E>       no repetition

Method of administration         1 <E>     i.v. bolus
```

The dialogue then returns to the CONTROL menu and option 2, `Set timings for run`, is chosen.

The questions are:

```
Enter length of run in h         3 <E>

number of results                30 <E>

times or interval                2 <E>      interval

enter interval in h              0.1 <E>
```

The CONTROL menu reappears and option 3, `Specify subject`, is entered. The dialogue is:

```
1 standard, 2 own subject        1 <E>      standard
```

The three essential specifications, necessary for starting a run, have now been made and when the CONTROL menu again appears, all the three markers will have gone; option 5, `Start run at zero time`, is now selected and on pressing `<E>`, a question asking for the type of primary display to be used appears.

```
Do you want the primary display to be

1) tabular, 2) graphical,

3) disposition diagram

4) slowed version of 3 ?        2<E>
```

The tabular display consists of six columns giving numerical details at each time point requested (Section 4.3, Table 2.3); the graphical display, which is chosen above for this run, is a broad range, five-cycle semilog plot of *C* against *t*; the layout of the disposition diagram is shown in Figure 2.5 and described in Section 4.3.

The semilog (semi because only one axis, the *C* axis, is logarithmic) is chosen in this case with the reply 2. The plot shows a broken horizontal line corresponding to the estimated minimum plasma concentration for drug activity; a full horizontal line shows the minimum concentration for drug toxicity.

The primary display graph has a five-cycle range to accommodate most needs for the different drugs available. It is usually desirable to produce a second plot with a narrower range of concentrations which you can either design yourself, or ask to have scaled automatically using the minimum C value and the number of log cycles represented in the stored results.

After the primary display is completed, on pressing <E>, the CONTROL menu again appears and option 7, `Display results`, is chosen. Subsequent dialogue is then:

```
Type of display              2 <E>      semilog plot

Minimum C                    <E>        automatic choice

Number of cycles             <E>        automatic choice
```

On pressing the final <E>, the axes appear followed rapidly by the plot displaying the already calculated results. In order to obtain a print-out of this plot as shown in *Figure 2.1*, the <PrtSc> key is pressed.

The first run is now complete.

When the print-out is finished, on pressing <E>, the DISPLAY sub-menu returns to the screen. Option 4, `No more displays`, is then chosen, the CONTROL menu now reappears and option 10, `Restart, different drug`, is selected to prepare for the second run of experiment 1, with thiopentone.

As shown in *Figure 2.1*, the log(C),t plot for gentamicin is almost linear, apart from the first point at 0.1 h. By 0.2 h the straight line is reached, indicating that the complete distribution volume is attained within 0.2 h of the dose being given.

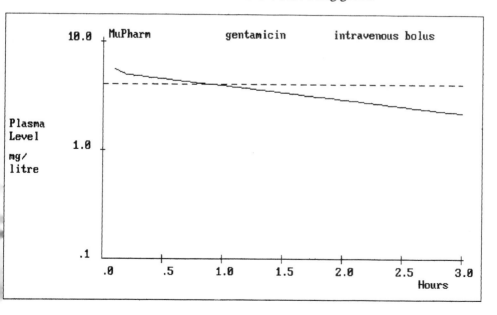

Press any key to continue

Figure 2.1 Gentamicin 120-mg i.v. bolus.

3.3.2 *Thiopentone*

The second part of the experiment is to repeat the run with thiopentone. This run only differs from that with gentamicin in the choice of drug and the size of the dose, 250 mg; details of the dialogue are summarized below.

```
DRUG SELECTION                    18 <E>    thiopentone
```

Since the timings and the subject are the same as for the previous study (with gentamicin), and we have not deleted this information, they do not have to be re-entered, though if it were necessary they could both be changed at this point.

When the CONTROL menu reappears there is only one marker, opposite option 1, indicating that this is the only option which must be re-entered.

The dialogue continues:

```
CONTROL                            1 <E>    prescription

DOSE AND METHOD

   Enter the dose in mg          250 <E>

   Multiple doses                  <E>      no

   Method                         1 <E>     i.v. bolus

CONTROL                           5 <E>     start at zero time

   Primary display                2         semilog plot
```

The run now commences with the five-cycle semilog display. When the plot is complete (3 h with results every 0.1 h), a better semilog plot is set up using the display option in the CONTROL menu. As with gentamicin, the automatic values for minimum C and number of cycles are chosen. <E> is pressed on completion of the run and the dialogue is:

```
CONTROL                            7 <E>    display

DISPLAY                            2 <E>    semilog plot

   Minimum concentration           <E>      automatic choice

   number of log cycles            <E>      automatic choice
```

The plot appears and may be printed out as before; the result is shown in *Figure 2.2*.

Experiment 1 is now complete and the user exits from the MuPharm program. Pressing <E> when print-out is completed brings back the DISPLAY sub-menu:

```
DISPLAY                    4 <E>      no more displays

CONTROL                   11 <E>      stop

Type your name for labelling output     giles
```

The last question is used to label the results-log with your name. This log is a tabular print-out of all the results obtained during a session. After the name is entered, execution reverts to the computer operating system.

The results-log may be displayed on the screen or printed using commands described in the implementation notes. The log remains until the next MuPharm run is started, at which point it is automatically overwritten.

The semilog C,t plot is shown in *Figure 2.2*. The shape of the plot is very different from that for gentamicin. The early points up to about 1 h lie on a curve well above the late time straight line, extended back to the axis. As discussed in Chapter 1, Section 5.2, a drug giving a semilog plot like this is said to show biphasic disposition kinetics.

The first, curved part of the graph in *Figure 2.2* is the alpha phase during which the drug is being distributed out from the plasma. The second, straight line part of the graph is the beta phase, during which the complete volume of distribution has been attained and the drug elimination proceeds as with gentamicin.

The transition between alpha and beta phases occurs at around 1 h after dose, indicating that the final distribution volume is not attained until this time.

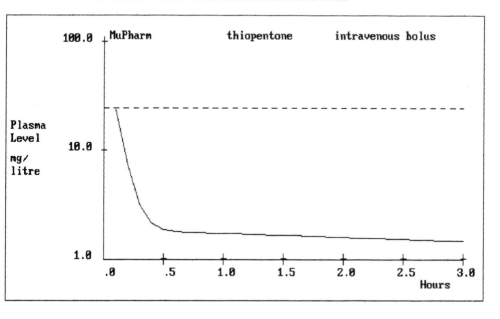

Press any key to continue

Figure 2.2 Thiopentone 250-mg i.v. bolus; biphasic semilog plot.

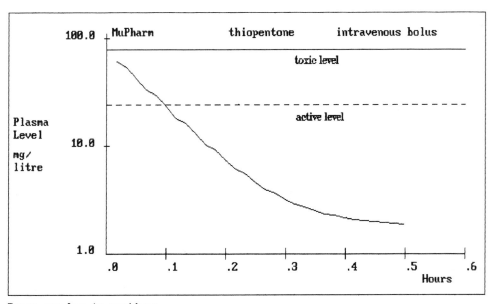

Figure 2.3 Thiopentone 250-mg i.v. bolus; short-acting anaesthetic effect.

The distribution of thiopentone is in fact quite complicated. The drug is highly soluble in lipids and there is rapid distribution to the brain, giving the anaesthetic effect which occurs in the alpha phase of the curve. Subsequently, the drug is distributed more slowly to muscle and to body fat. This further distribution causes the sharp fall of plasma concentrations in the alpha phase.

The onset of anaesthesia with thiopentone is within seconds of the dose and the duration is about 5 min. These results are seen in the time-expanded plot shown in *Figure 2.3*. To obtain this plot a run was set up of 0.5 h duration and with 30 results at 0.0166-h, i.e. 1-min, intervals.

3.4 Conclusions from experiment 1

Gentamicin rapidly reaches the complete volume of distribution, while thiopentone gives a biphasic semilog plot indicating a slower attainment of this complete volume. The initial rapid distribution of thiopentone to the brain is followed by a slower distribution to muscle and lipid, resulting in the curved semilog plot.

4. EXPERIMENT 2: TO DETERMINE PHARMACOKINETIC PARAMETERS FOLLOWING INTRAVENOUS INFUSIONS OF AMPICILLIN AND THEOPHYLLINE

4.1 Objectives

The objectives of this experiment are to determine the plasma half-life for ampicillin and the areas under the C,t curves for both drugs, and to evaluate the volumes of distribution and total clearances. The renal clearances are calculated from the values of plasma concentration and the amount of drug excreted in the urine, given in the tables of numerical results. These values are obtained by printing out the results-log after the experiment has been completed.

The two drugs chosen contrast with one another in that ampicillin, an antibiotic, is rapidly eliminated with a half-life of around 1.5 h, while theophylline, a drug used to treat asthma, has a longer half-life of around 9 h.

The subject used is the standard one in the simulation model.

4.2 Plan for experiment 2

In order to estimate the plasma half-life for ampicillin, a run is set up with a dose of 250 mg i.v. bolus. The half-life is short and so a run time of 6 h with 12 results at 0.5-h intervals is specified. The primary display chosen is the semilog plot. After this is completed, a semilog graph with fewer log cycles is plotted from the stored results.

The dose used in the run for the calculation of area is 250 mg i.v. infusion over 0.5 h. An i.v. bolus dose is unsuitable because of the high and rapidly changing initial concentrations. For area determinations following i.v. dose, both in reality and in the simulation model, the i.v. infusion method is best used. In the simulation model, a request for a calculation of area is refused when the method of administration is i.v. bolus and a message is displayed, recommending you to use i.v. infusion.

The approximate half-lives for the drugs in the simulation program are given in Appendix II. The length of the run should be at least three half-lives, with results close together at first.

The half-life of ampicillin is about 1.5 h and so a run length for area determination of 8 h is more than sufficient. Eleven results are specified, at 0.25, 0.5, 0.75, 1, 1.25, 1.5, 2, 3, 4, 6 and 8 h.

The half-life for theophylline is around 9 h, a dose of 200 mg is given as an i.v. infusion over 0.5 h and a run of 36 h is made with 16 results recorded; the first 11 are as for ampicillin, the remaining five results are at 12, 18, 24, 30 and 36h.

For the area calculation runs, the disposition diagram is chosen as the primary display, followed by selecting the area calculation and then the C,t plots.

At the end of the experiment, the results-log is printed out to obtain the tables of numerical values. Instructions for the printing are contained in the implementation notes.

4.3 Runs and results

4.3.1 Ampicillin

The dialogue for the first run, which is for determining half-life only and so does not require area calculations, is set out below.

Summary of dialogue

```
DRUG                     1 <E>      ampicillin

CONTROL                  1 <E>      prescribe drug
```

```
DOSE AND METHOD

    dose, mg                   250 <E>

    multiple doses             <E>

    method of admin            1 <E>      i.v. bolus

CONTROL                        2 <E>      set run

SET RUN

    length of run h            6 <E>

    number of results          12 <E>

    times or interval          2 <E>      interval

    enter interval             0.5 <E>

CONTROL                        3 <E>      subject

SUBJECT

    1 standard, 2 own          1 <E>

CONTROL                        5 <E>      start zero time

    Primary display            2 <E>      semilog plot
```
At the end of the run:
```
                               <E>

CONTROL                        7 <E>      display

DISPLAY

    type                       2 <E>      semilog plot

    minimum C                  <E>        automatic

    number of cycles           <E>        automatic

                               <PrtSc>
```
After the display has been printed:

```
                               <E>

DISPLAY                        4 <E>      no more displays

CONTROL                        9 <E>      restart same drug
```

The program is then ready for the next run with ampicillin.

The semilog plot for ampicillin in *Figure 2.4* shows that there is a biphasic effect. The beta phase starts at 1 h and so the triangle *PQR* (Chapter 1, Section 4.3) is drawn with *PQ* at 3 h and *R* at 5 h.

In order to find the length of *PQ* in log units, it is measured in millimetres and is divided by the length of the log unit in millimetres. This latter is the distance between any two concentrations differing by a factor of 10 on the vertical axis.

From *Figure 2.4*, $PQ = 0.384$ log units, $QR = 2$ h, therefore the elimination rate constant is

$$k = 2.3 \times 0.384/2 = 0.442 \text{ h}^{-1}$$

The half-life is then:

$$t_{1/2} = 0.693/0.442 = 1.57 \text{ h}$$

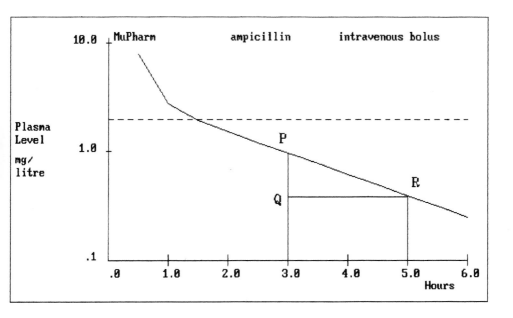

Press any key to continue

Figure 2.4 Ampicillin 250-mg i.v. bolus; half-life estimation.

An alternative method for determining k and $t_{1/2}$ is to use the numerical C,t values. At least three pairs which are in the straight line region of the semilog plot are taken and a linear regression analysis is used to estimate the slope of the $\ln(C),t$ line. Numerical values of the plasma concentrations are obtained from a print-out of the results-log at the end of the experiment.

In the simulation model dialogue, option 8 on the CONTROL menu, Estimate area under C,t plot, performs the regression calculation on the last three data points, which should be in the straight line region of the semilog plot, and displays the values of elimination constant and plasma half-life. The value of $t_{1/2}$ found in the next run by this method is 1.53 h.

The details for setting up the second ampicillin run are set out below.

Summary of dialogue

CONTROL	1 <E>	prescribe drug
DOSE AND METHOD		
dose, mg	250 <E>	
multiple doses	<E>	
method of admin	2 <E>	i.v. infusion
duration 1st inf, h	0.5 <E>	
2nd infusion	<E>	no
CONTROL	2 <E>	set run
SET RUN		
length of run h	8 <E>	
number of results	11 <E>	
times or interval	1 <E>	times
enter times	0.25 <E> 0.5 <E> 0.75 <E>	
	1 <E> 1.25 <E> 1.5 <E>	
	2 <E> 3 <E> 4 <E> 6 <E>	
	8 <E>	

```
CONTROL                    3 <E>     subject

SUBJECT

  1 standard, 2 own        1 <E>

CONTROL                    5 <E>     start zero time

  Primary display          3 <E>     disposition

                                     diagram

                           <PrtSc>
```

At the end of the printing the area calculation is selected and the results appear on the screen and are also recorded in the results-log.

```
                           <E>

CONTROL                    8 <E>     area calculation
```
The C,t plot is then selected.

```
                           <E>

CONTROL                    7 <E>     display

DISPLAY

  type                     1 <E>     C,t plot

                           <PrtSc>
```
After the display has been printed:

```
                           <E>

DISPLAY                    4 <E>     no more displays

CONTROL                   10 <E>     restart new drug
```

The next run, which is with theophylline, may then be set up.

The disposition diagram. The disposition diagram, chosen as the primary display in this run, is shown in *Figure 2.5*. It consists of five boxes, a small-scale five-cycle semilog C,t plot, the same as that in the primary graphical display, a digital clock showing time after the start of the run and details of the prescription.

In all the boxes the top of the black area shows the proportion of the total dose which is in that box; this proportion is shown on the scale on the side of the box. The top of the stippled area shows the maximum filling of the box during the run. The levels move as the simulation progresses.

The *residual dose* box fills completely for doses given by the i.v. route. With i.v. bolus the whole dose then passes rapidly into the *plasma* box; in the plasma box the proportion of total dose is read directly from the scale, for the i.v. route. For the oral and i.m. routes, the proportion in this box is small and is therefore multiplied by 10, the full scale value for these two routes is therefore 0.1.

When the drug is given as an i.v. infusion, the residual dose box empties into the plasma gradually, according to the infusion rate.

The plasma amount starts to decrease as the drug enters the other three boxes. In the *outer distribution* box, the level at first rises to a maximum and then falls as the plasma level falls. The stippled area indicates the maximum filling reached.

In the *metabolism* box, the black area continues to rise throughout the run, as it does in the *excretion* (urinary) box. The heights in these two boxes indicate the relative importance of these two elimination pathways.

When a drug is given by the oral route (Chapter 3, Section 2.3, Figure 3.2), the residual dose box does not usually fill completely and the white area at the top represents the proportion of the dose which is not available for absorption into the plasma. The black level in this box drops as drug is absorbed into the plasma, leaving the stippled area to show the maximum filling of the box. Drug then proceeds to the three disposition boxes. The i.m. route gives similar results.

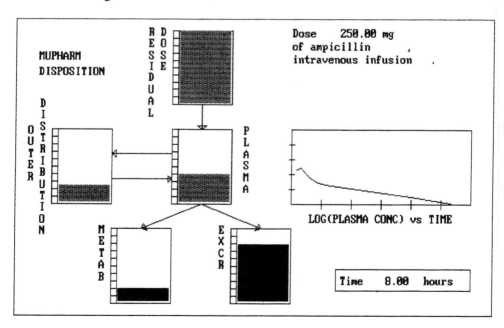

Press any key to continue

Figure 2.5 Ampicillin; disposition diagram at 8 h.

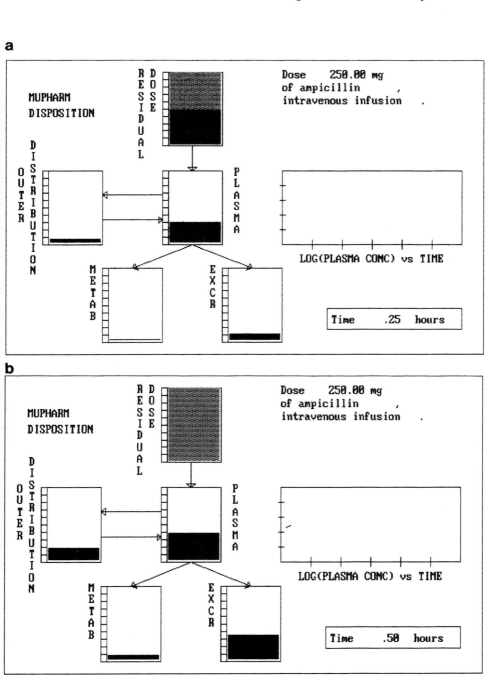

Figure 2.6 Ampicillin at: (a) 0.25 h; (b) 0.5 h

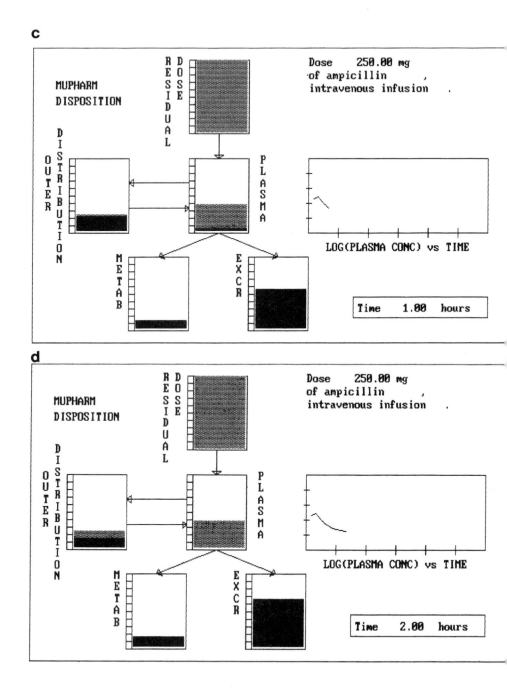

Figure 2.6 Ampicillin at: (c) 1 h; (d) 2 h

With short time intervals, the changes in the diagram occur rapidly, and on faster micro-computers it is desirable to be able to slow them down. A complete speed control is available by changing the iteration interval (Appendix VIII) for the calculations. When the prescription, run and subject details have been entered, option 4 on the CONTROL menu is chosen, giving the CHANGE sub-menu. Option 1 then enables the iteration interval to be changed. This interval is normally 0.01 h, changing it to 0.001 h gives a suitably slow movement in the disposition diagram. As a result of choosing option 4 for the primary display, the iteration time is reduced automatically by a factor of 10 and then restored to its previous value on completion of the run.

The results in *Figure 2.5* show that at the end of 8 h, the plasma and outer distribution volume boxes are empty, the metabolism box is filled to the 0.2 mark while the excretion box is filled almost to 0.8. Metabolism is therefore a lesser route for the elimination of ampicillin.

The progress of the disposition may be followed by printing out the diagrams obtained by making a series of shorter runs.

Results of such 'snapshots' for the ampicillin run are shown in *Figure 2.6*. As with *Figure 2.5*, the dose is 250 mg ampicillin, i.v. infusion over 0.5 h with the standard subject, C values are recorded at 0.25-h intervals.

In *Figure 2.6a* the run length is 0.25 h and it is seen that the residual dose box is half emptied (total infusion time 0.5 h); the plasma box partly filled; the outer distribution and excretion boxes are beginning to fill.

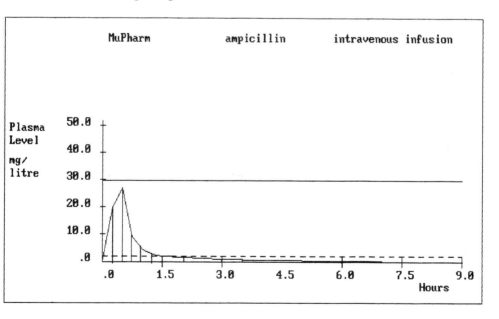

Press any key to continue

Figure 2.7 Ampicillin 250-mg/0.5-h i.v. infusion, area estimation.

For *Figure 2.6b* the run length is 0.5 h and the residual dose box has now emptied; the plasma and the outer distribution proportions have increased; the excretion has increased substantially in accordance with the short half-life of ampicillin; the proportion in the metabolism box is growing slowly.

In *Figure 2.6c* the run length is 1 h, the plasma proportion has now dropped markedly, the outer disposition level has also dropped, leaving the stippled area to indicate the maximum level attained; excretion and metabolism levels have both increased.

Figure 2.6d is for a run length of 2 h, plasma and outer disposition are emptying and much of the drug has been excreted or metabolized. The changes then continue in the same way until at 8 h, as shown in *Figure 2.5*, all the boxes except metabolism and excretion are empty.

The C,t plot of the results of the area run with ampicillin is shown in *Figure 2.7*. The area under the curve may be assessed by drawing vertical lines at each data point, as shown in the figure, calculating the areas of each strip (equal to base multiplied by mean height) and adding the strip areas together (Chapter 1, Section 9.1). Note that this area is the area under the C,t curve, not the area under a semilog plot. The latter area cannot be defined from $C = 0$ and is not used in any subsequent calculations.

The summation of strip areas is a tedious arithmetical operation and so a routine has been included in the simulation program to perform the calculation. This routine is available by selecting option 8 on the CONTROL menu.

The importance of the area under the C,t curve in pharmacokinetics, reflecting the amount of drug which has passed through the plasma, has been discussed in Chapter 1, Section 9.3.

Table 2.3 Ampicillin, area estimation.

```
**********MUPHARM RESULTS-LOG**********

Dose     250.00 mg of ampicillin        intravenous infusion
1st infusion     .50 h, 2nd infusion     .00 mg/h for     .00 h

Numerical Details
```

time,h	cp,mg/l	xd,mg	xm,mg	xu,mg	respons
.25	20.52	16.11	6.94	28.06	++
.50	27.14	45.73	21.13	85.43	++
.75	9.40	60.15	30.94	125.09	+
1.00	4.42	58.88	34.74	140.48	+
1.25	2.88	53.96	36.82	148.86	+
1.50	2.29	48.56	38.31	154.90	+
2.00	1.73	38.83	40.63	164.29	−
3.00	1.10	24.70	43.89	177.46	−
4.00	.70	15.70	45.96	185.83	−
6.00	.28	6.35	48.11	194.53	−
8.00	.11	2.57	48.98	198.04	−

```
AREA UNDER THE CURVE

The late time elimination constant is    .4529 1/h
The half life based on the last 3 points is     1.53 h
The extrapolation term is      .25 hour.mg/litre
The estimate of total area is      21.32 hour.mg/litre
```

For the estimation of other pharmacokinetic parameters it is necessary to know the total area under the C,t curve to infinite time, found by using the extrapolation term (Chapter 1, Section 9.2 and Appendix I, Section 2.2).

If the area up to time t_n is area_n, the total area is area_T and the concentration at time t_n is C_n and the late time elimination constant is k:

$$\text{area}_T = \text{area}_n + C_n/k$$

The estimate of area is obtained by choosing option 8 on the CONTROL menu. The elimination rate constant and the late time plasma half-life, based on a regression analysis of the last three $\ln(C),t$ values in the data, the area extrapolation term and the total area are then calculated and the values of these four quantities are displayed.

Numerical results from this run are shown in *Table 2.3*, which comes from the results-log printed out at the end of the experiment; if option 8 has been chosen, the parameter estimates from the area calculation are listed at the end of the table.

When a table of numerical values is required (except when decisions for the next run have to be based on the results), it is preferable to take it from the results-log since this log gives details of the prescription, the subject and any factor changes which have been made.

The table of results has six columns; the first is time in hours; the second is plasma concentration either in mg/l or in µg/l as shown by the heading; the third is the amount of drug currently distributed outside the plasma in mg; the fourth is the cumulative amount metabolized in mg; the fifth is the cumulative amount eliminated in the urine in mg; the sixth is the estimated subject response to the drug.

The response is denoted by '−' for inactive; '+' for active; '++' for an active response with a plasma concentration C more than half-way to the minimum toxic level; 'toxicity' for C in the toxic range; 'death' if C reaches the lethal level. In the event of death, the calculation stops and a message is printed out.

The active, toxic and lethal levels are set by drug factors 18, 16 and 17 (see Chapter 4 for details of changing factors and Appendix II for values of the three levels for the 20 drugs) and may be changed by the user. They are only approximate indications of the expected drug responses.

Late time elimination rate constant, half-life and total area. From the area calculations listed in the results-log, the late time elimination rate constant for ampicillin is $0.453 \, \text{h}^{-1}$ and the half-life is 1.53 h. The total area is 21.3 h mg/l with an extrapolation term of 0.25 h mg/l, therefore the run has been continued long enough for the extrapolation term to be small compared with the total area.

Apparent volume of distribution. The apparent volume of distribution of a drug can be estimated from the total area under the C,t curve by means of the equation (Chapter 1, Section 9.5, equation 1.9)

$$F \times D = k \times V \times \text{area}_T$$

F is the bioavailability (Chapter 1, Section 9.4) which is 1.0 for the i.v. route; D is the dose in mg; k is the elimination rate constant in h^{-1}; V is the apparent final volume of distribution in litres; area_T is the total area under the C,t curve in h mg/l.

The above equation only applies to drugs which have first-order disposition. If there is capacity-limited metabolism, as with phenytoin, it is no longer valid except at very low doses (see Chapter 7).

From this equation the apparent volume of distribution is calculated directly:

$$V = D/(k \times \text{area}_T) = 250/(0.453 \times 21.3) = 25.9 \text{ l}$$

This volume, which includes the plasma volume, is low compared with the total body water of a 70-kg subject (of the order of 40 l).

The indication is that ampicillin, which is a highly polar, water-soluble drug, is not widely distributed.

Renal clearance. Renal clearance is the rate of elimination of a drug in the urine in mg/ h, divided by the mean plasma concentration of the drug over the period used to measure the elimination rate (Chapter 1, Section 10.2, equation 1.11):

$$Cl_r = \text{rate}(X)_u(\text{mg/h})/C_{\text{mean}}(\text{mg/l}) \text{ l/h}$$

The importance of clearance is that if the urinary elimination is first order, as it is for most drugs, the clearance is constant for a given subject, independent of dose and of plasma level (see Appendix I, Section 4.1). This constant clearance can then be used to assess the rate of urinary elimination in mg/h at any given plasma concentration.

The renal clearance for ampicillin can be calculated from the numerical results in *Table 2.3*. An interval well after the end of the infusion time is chosen. Since C varies rapidly with t, a short interval, between 3 and 4 h, is used.

The mean rate of urinary excretion over this interval is calculated from the difference in the column 5 values in the table of results (*Table 2.3*), of the cumulative amount excreted in the urine X_u:

$$\text{rate}(X)_u = 185.83 - 177.46 = 8.37 \text{ mg/h}$$

The mean plasma concentration over the interval is

$$C_{\text{mean}} = (1.10 + 0.70)/2 = 0.9 \text{ mg/l}$$

The renal clearance is therefore

$$Cl_r = \text{rate}(X)_u/C_{\text{mean}} = 8.37/0.9 = 9.3 \text{ l/h}$$

The renal clearance of a drug may be compared with the glomerular filtration rate *GFR* (Chapter 1, Section 7.2) for the subject. For the standard subject in the model the value of *GFR* is 7.5 l/h. The fact that the renal clearance of ampicillin is larger indicates that there is an active transfer of the drug to the filtrate from the plasma in the renal tubules, in addition to the glomerular filtration.

Total clearance. By analogy with renal clearance, the concept of total clearance Cl_T has been defined in Chapter 1, Section 10.3 as

$$Cl_T = \text{rate}(X)_{e,\text{mean}}/C_{\text{mean}} = F \times D/\text{area}_T \text{ l/h}$$

An alternative expression for Cl_T may be derived from Chapter 1, equation (1.9):

$$F \times D = k \times V \times \text{area}_T \quad \text{therefore} \quad F \times D/\text{area}_T = k \times V$$

$$Cl_T = F \times D/\text{area}_T = k \times V$$

If the elimination is first-order, Cl_T is constant and independent of dose since both k and V are constants for a given subject; with drugs with capacity-limited metabolism (Chapter 7), this is not correct since the apparent elimination rate constant k decreases as C increases, causing a reduction in clearance at high concentrations.

When the dose is given by the i.v. route, the bioavailability F is 1.0.

The total clearance for ampicillin is therefore

$$Cl_T = D/\text{area}_T = 250/21.3 = 11.7 \text{ l/h}$$

Hepatic clearance (Chapter 1, Section 10.4). The difference between Cl_T and Cl_r may be considered to be the hepatic clearance, Cl_h. The estimated hepatic clearance for ampicillin is:

$$Cl_h = Cl_T - Cl_r = 11.7 - 9.3 = 2.4 \text{ l/h}$$

Comparison of Cl_h and Cl_r shows that ampicillin is mainly cleared as unchanged drug in the urine. Metabolism is a smaller elimination pathway, as is seen in the disposition diagram (*Figure 2.5*).

4.3.2 Theophylline

The run to determine the area under the C,t curve for theophylline is set up according to the plan in Section 4.2. Since this run follows on from the ampicillin run, there is no need to reselect the subject; both prescription and run details have to be altered.

Summary of dialogue

DRUG	14 <E>	theophylline
CONTROL	1 <E>	prescribe drug
DOSE AND METHOD		
dose, mg	200 <E>	
multiple doses	<E>	no
method of admin	2 <E>	i.v. infusion
duration infusion h	0.5 <E>	
second infusion	<E>	no
CONTROL	2 <E>	set run

```
SET RUN

    length of run h              36 <E>

    number of results           16 <E>

    times or interval           1 <E>        specify times

    enter times                 0.25 <E> 0.5 <E> 0.75 <E>

                                 1 <E> 1.25 <E> 1.5 <E>

                                 2 <E> 3 <E> 4 <E>

                                 6 <E> 8 <E> 12 <E>

                                 18 <E> 24 <E> 30 <E>

                                 36 <E>

CONTROL                          5 <E>        start zero time

    primary display             3 <E>        disposition
                                              diagram

                                 <PrtSc>
```

At the end of the printing the area calculation is selected:

```
                                 <E>

CONTROL                          8 <E>        area calculation
```

After the area results have been displayed and recorded automatically on the results-log, the *C,t* plot is selected:

```
                                 <E>

CONTROL                          7 <E>        display

DISPLAY

    type                        1 <E>        C,t plot

                                 <PrtSc>
```

After the display has been printed the simulation session is stopped:

```
                           <E>

DISPLAY                    4 <E>      no more displays

CONTROL                    11 <E>     stop

Type your name for labelling print-out giles
```

At this stage the results-log may be printed out.

Disposition diagram. Figure 2.8 shows that at the end of 36 h there are negligible amounts of theophylline left in both the plasma and the outer distribution volume. In contrast to ampicillin, it is the metabolism box that is almost full while the urinary excretion of unchanged drug is a minor route.

Elimination constant and plasma half-life. From the area calculation recorded in the results-log shown in *Table 2.4*, the late time elimination constant is 0.0801 h^{-1} and the corresponding plasma half-life is 8.65 h.

Area. The plot from which the area would be estimated by the trapezium method is shown in *Figure 2.9*.

From *Table 2.4* the value of area$_T$ is 71.3 h mg/l. The run has been continued long enough to make the extrapolation term, 3.59 h mg/l, a relatively small proportion of area$_T$.

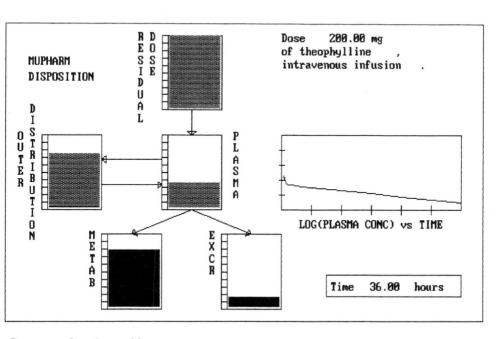

Press any key to continue

Figure 2.8 Theophylline, disposition diagram.

L. Saunders, D. Ingram and S. H. D. Jackson

Apparent volume of distribution. The apparent volume of distribution is given by rearranging equation (1.9):

$$V = D/(k \times \text{area}_T) = 200/(0.0801 \times 71.3) = 35.0\ \text{l}$$

This volume is larger than that for ampicillin, indicating that theophylline is distributed somewhat more widely.

Renal clearance. The renal clearance of theophylline is calculated from the data in *Table 2.4*, taking the 6- to 8-h values of urinary excretion and plasma concentration:

$$\text{rate}(X)_u = (17.91 - 15.07)/2 = 1.42\ \text{mg/h}$$

$$C_{\text{mean}} = (3.18 + 2.71)/2 = 2.95\ \text{mg/l}$$

$$Cl_r = \text{rate}(X)_u/C_{\text{mean}} = 1.42/2.95 = 0.48\ \text{l/h}$$

This value is very much less than the glomerular filtration rate.

Total clearance. The total clearance of theophylline is:

$$Cl_T = D/\text{area}_T = 200/71.3 = 2.81\ \text{l/h}$$

Table 2.4 Theophylline, area.

```
**********MUPHARM RESULTS-LOG**********

Dose       200.00 mg of theophylline      intravenous infusion
1st infusion      .50 h, 2nd infusion      .00 mg/h for      .00 h

Numerical Details

time,h     cp,mg/l      xd,mg        xm,mg        xu,mg      respons
   .25      15.32        38.49         5.28         1.09      +
   .50      20.24       108.03        15.82         3.27      ++
   .75       7.81       143.87        23.23         4.80      +
  1.00       5.32       148.38        26.91         5.56      +
  1.25       4.76       146.86        29.83         6.17      -
  1.50       4.58       144.22        32.56         6.73      -
  2.00       4.38       138.62        37.80         7.82      -
  3.00       4.04       127.95        47.65         9.85      -
  4.00       3.73       118.10        56.74        11.73      -
  6.00       3.18       100.61        72.88        15.07      -
  8.00       2.71        85.72        86.62        17.91      -
 12.00       1.97        62.21       108.32        22.40      -
 18.00       1.22        38.47       130.23        26.93      -
 24.00        .75        23.79       143.78        29.73      -
 30.00        .46        14.71       152.16        31.46      -
 36.00        .29         9.09       157.34        32.53      -

AREA UNDER THE CURVE

The late time elimination constant is   .0801 1/h
The half life based on the last 3 points is      8.65 h
The extrapolation term is      3.59 hour.mg/litre
The estimate of total area is      71.34 hour.mg/litre
```

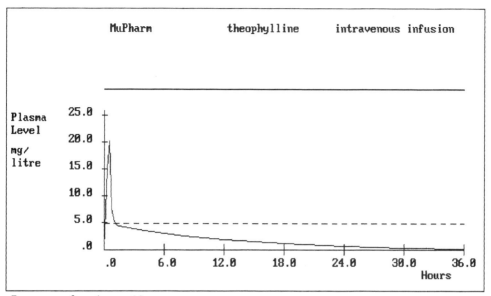

Press any key to continue
Figure 2.9 Theophylline 200-mg/0.5-h i.v. infusion.

Hepatic clearance. An estimate of hepatic clearance is:

$$Cl_h = 2.81 - 0.48 = 2.33 \text{ l/h}$$

Metabolism is therefore the principal clearance mechanism for theophylline, with urinary excretion as a lesser route of elimination — a result which is also shown in the disposition diagram.

4.4 Conclusions from experiment 2

Ampicillin and theophylline possess contrasting physical and pharmacokinetic properties. Ampicillin is a highly polar, water-soluble acid which has a low solubility in lipid solvents such as ether and chloroform, leading to a relatively small apparent volume of distribution. It is only minimally bound to plasma proteins (fraction bound 0.18) and is rapidly eliminated due to specific transfer in the tubules. The disposition diagram and the relative values of renal and hepatic clearances show that metabolism is a lesser route for the elimination of ampicillin.

Theophylline is a weak acid which is sparingly soluble in water and in lipid solvents, with a larger apparent volume of distribution than that for ampicillin. The disposition diagram and the renal and hepatic clearances show that theophylline is mainly eliminated by metabolism.

5. PROBLEMS

1.   From the C,t data in *Tables 2.3* and *2.4*, use the trapezium method to estimate area values for ampicillin and theophylline and compare them with the values from the area calculations in the simulation program.

2. Using runs in the simulation model similar to those in Chapter 2, evaluate the pharmacokinetic parameters for single i.v. doses of oxprenolol (see Appendix II for properties) given to the standard subject. Suitable doses are 20 mg i.v. bolus and 20 mg i.v. infusion over 0.5 h.

CHAPTER 3

Single Oral and Intramuscular Dose Experiments to Determine Pharmacokinetic Parameters. Studies with Ampicillin, Nortriptyline and Gentamicin

1. PARAMETERS FOR THE ORAL ROUTE

Use of the oral route of administration gives rise to some new characteristic features of observed drug kinetics. These features are quantified in terms of further pharmacokinetic parameters described in the following sections, which are supplementary to those considered in Chapter 2, Section 1.

1.1 Lag time, t_{lag}

Lag time is the period following oral dose before a detectable amount of drug appears in the plasma; its length depends on the dosage form and the sensitivity of the assay.

Solutions and suspensions give rapid drug uptake and a negligible lag time. Compressed tablets and capsules usually give lag times of a fraction of an hour, while sustained release preparations may give lag times of one hour or more.

1.2 Maximum concentration and time of maximum, C_{max} and t_{max}

The relatively slow absorption from oral doses gives a C,t plot showing a maximum plasma concentration C_{max}, as in *Figure 3.1*. It is difficult to estimate an absorption rate constant from the data owing to interference between absorption and distribution. With different formulations of the same drug dose, C_{max} and the time after dose at which it occurs, t_{max}, are used to compare rates of absorption.

1.3 Bioavailability, F

The bioavailability of a drug from an oral dose is the fraction of the dose which reaches the plasma intact. This fraction is often less than 1.0 due to incomplete absorption from the dosage form and to first-pass metabolism (Chapter 1, Section 6.5)

The total area under a C,t curve is a measure of the amount of drug which has passed through the plasma of the subject (Chapter 1, Section 9.3 and Appendix I, Section 2.1). The bioavailability, F (Chapter 1, Section 9.4), is estimated as the ratio of the total area under the C,t curve when a dose D is given by the oral route, to the total area when the same dose is given to the same subject by i.v. infusion.

F is defined by the equation

$$F = \text{area}_T(D,\text{oral})/\text{area}_T(D,\text{i.v.})$$

In practice, with more toxic drugs, the i.v. dose is reduced so as to avoid transient toxic effects resulting from the high initial concentrations of the drug. Bioavailability is only meaningful for drugs having first-order disposition kinetics, so that area_T is proportional to dose. If the oral dose is D_2 and the i.v. dose is D_1, then on this proportionality basis, the estimated area for an i.v. dose of D_2 is

$$\text{area}_T(D_2,\text{i.v.}) = \text{area}_T(D_1,\text{i.v.}) \times D_2/D_1$$

and the bioavailabilty is

$$F = \text{area}_T(D_2,\text{oral})/[(D_2/D_1) \times \text{area}_T(D_1,\text{i.v.})]$$

(3.1)

Intravenous doses are taken up completely into the plasma and so this ratio measures the fraction of the oral dose which reaches the plasma intact.

1.4 Fraction of the dose absorbed, F_a

Many drugs are incompletely absorbed from an oral dose. There may also be significant transport of a drug in the bile, to excretion in the faeces. Unless it undergoes hepatic circulation and is reabsorbed, drug eliminated through the bile does not reach the main plasma volume and it may therefore be included in the fraction of dose not absorbed.

The fraction absorbed from the dose into the main plasma volume (including drug metabolized in the first pass and subsequently) is assessed from urinary excretion studies. A run is continued until almost all the drug has been eliminated (more than five half-lives). The total sum of all the drug excreted and metabolized may be taken as the total amount of drug which has reached the plasma.

In practice, it is difficult to measure the total amount of drug metabolized, though isotope studies can be helpful. With some drugs, excretion pathways other than the urine may be important.

In the simplified situation in the model, F_a may be assessed as the sum of the cumulative amounts which have been metabolized or excreted unchanged in the urine in a run long enough to give total elimination of the drug, divided by the dose given.

1.5 Hepatic extraction ratio, E

The fraction of the amount of drug absorbed from an oral dose which is metabolized in the first pass through the liver is called the hepatic extraction ratio, E. As shown in Chapter 1, equation (1.5):

$$E = 1 - F/F_a$$

where F_a and F may be determined in the simulation model as described above. In reality, determining F_a for drugs which undergo first-pass metabolism may be difficult.

2. EXPERIMENT 3: TO DETERMINE PARAMETERS FOLLOWING ORAL DOSES WITH AMPICILLIN AND NORTRIPTYLINE

2.1 Objectives

The objectives of this experiment are to assess the oral dose parameters for ampicillin and nortriptyline, drugs which show contrasting pharmacokinetic behaviour. Ampicillin has already been studied by the i.v. route in experiment 2 (Chapter 2, Section 4). The i.v. area result from that study is used to assess the bioavailability from an oral dose.

2.2 Plan of the experiment

The first three oral dose parameters, t_{lag}, C_{max} and t_{max}, may be determined together, from the results of a short run with frequent recording of C values. A run time of 3 h with results every 0.25 h is used for both drugs; for ampicillin, a dose of 1000 mg is given and for nortriptyline the dose is 50 mg. The primary display is the semilog plot and a further C,t plot is selected; for nortriptyline, the primary display chosen is the disposition diagram.

Only a run for the oral dose area estimation is required for the bioavailability assessment with ampicillin. The run is set up as in Chapter 2, Section 4.3, with an oral dose of 1000 mg. The run time is 8 h with the 11 results at the same times as those used in the i.v. infusion run. The primary display is the disposition diagram, followed by selection of the area calculation and then by a C,t plot.

To determine the fractions absorbed, F_a, runs of more than five half-lives are required. In these runs, extended intervals between results may be used since it is only the final, cumulative values of the amounts metabolized and excreted, X_m and X_u, which are required. The option for tables of results is chosen for the primary displays so that the numerical results may be checked and the runs continued for further periods if elimination is not complete. A run time of 24 h with results every 6 h is suitable for ampicillin, the same final values would be obtained with a single set of results at 24 h but some intermediate results are useful for checking for complete elimination.

To determine the bioavailability of nortriptyline, both i.v. infusion and oral dose runs need to be made. A suitable dose for the oral route is 50 mg with a smaller dose of 10 mg used for the i.v. infusion, so as to avoid transient toxic effects. The approximate half-life is 24 h (Appendix II) and so runs of 72 h are set up, each with 17 results at the following times in hours.

0.25   0.5   0.75   1   1.25 1.5   2   3   4   6   8   12   24   36   48   60   72

To determine the fraction absorbed for nortriptyline a run of 144 h is used, with results every 24 h.

2.3 **Runs and results**

2.3.1 *Ampicillin*

The first ampicillin study is carried out to determine the three parameters associated with absorption, a therapeutic level, oral dose of 1000 mg is used; the run length is 3 h with 12 results at 0.25-h intervals.

Summary of dialogue

```
DRUG                        1 <E>      ampicillin

CONTROL                     1 <E>      prescribe drug

DOSE AND METHOD

    dose, mg                1000 <E>

    multiple doses          <E>        no

    method of admin         3 <E>      oral

CONTROL                     2 <E>      set run

SET RUN

    length of run h         3 <E>

    number of results       12 <E>

    times or interval       2 <E>      fixed interval

    enter interval          0.25 <E>

CONTROL                     3 <E>      subject

SUBJECT

    1 standard, 2 own       1 <E>

CONTROL                     5 <E>      start zero time

    primary display         2 <E>      semilog plot
```

At the end of the run:

	<E>	
CONTROL	7 <E>	display

DISPLAY

type	1 <E>	C,t plot
	<PrtSc>	

After the display has been printed:

	<E>	
DISPLAY	4 <E>	no more displays
CONTROL	9 <E>	restart same drug

The program is left ready for the next run with ampicillin.

The C,t results are shown in *Figure 3.1*. In order to find t_{lag}, the plot is produced to cut the time axis. The time at the point of intersection, if positive, is taken as the lag time. If the intercept is found to be negative, the lag time is taken as zero.

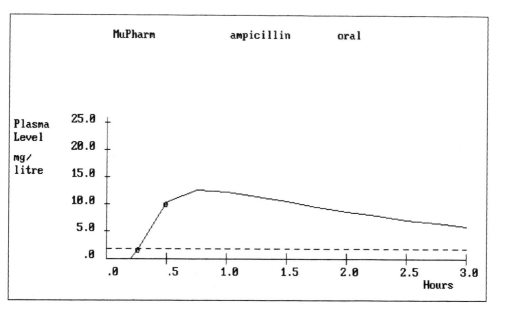

Press any key to continue

Figure 3.1 Ampicillin 1000 mg oral, short run.

67

From *Figure 3.1*, t_{lag} is 0.23 h. C_{max} and t_{max} are estimated as C_{max} = 12.8 mg/l, t_{max} = 0.75 h.

The next ampicillin run is designed for the determination of area$_T$(1000 mg,oral); the oral dose of 1000 mg is given to the standard subject and, since the dialogue is continued from the previous run, the dose and subject do not have to be re-entered. The summary of the dialogue for setting up the run is as follows.

Summary of dialogue

```
CONTROL                        2 <E>     set run

SET RUN

    length of run h            8 <E>

    number of results          11 <E>

    times or interval          1 <E>     specify times

    enter each time            0.25 <E> 0.5 <E> 0.75 <E>

                               1 <E> 1.25 <E> 1.5 <E>

                               2 <E> 3 <E> 4 <E>

                               6 <E> 8 <E>

CONTROL                        5 <E>     start zero time

    primary display            3 <E>     disposition

                                         diagram

                               <PrtSc>
```

At the end of the print-out, the area determination is chosen followed by the choice of a *C,t* plot.

```
                               <E>

CONTROL                        8 <E>     area
```

After noting the area, the elimination rate constant and the half-life from the screen:

```
                               <E>

CONTROL                        7 <E>     display
```

```
DISPLAY

    type                        1 <E>     C,t plot

                                <PrtSc>
```

After the display has been printed:

```
                                <E>

DISPLAY                         4 <E>     no more displays

CONTROL                         9 <E>     restart same drug
```

The program is left ready for the next run with ampicillin.

The disposition diagram for oral ampicillin 8 h after dose is shown in *Figure 3.2*. The blank space at the top of the residual dose box shows that only half the dose is available for absorption. Both plasma and outer distribution boxes are empty, indicating substantially complete elimination at 8 h. As with the i.v. route (*Figure 2.5*), elimination is mainly by urinary excretion of unchanged drug.

The C,t results are shown graphically in *Figure 3.3* and the detailed numerical values taken from the results-log printed out at the end of this experiment are given in *Table 3.1*.

Plasma half-life. The value of the elimination rate constant k from *Table 3.1*, is 0.418 h^{-1}. The half-life $t_{1/2}$ is 1.66 h, higher than the value of 1.53 h obtained in the i.v. infusion run (Chapter 2, Section 4.3). This difference is due to continuing absorption during the later stages of the short run.

Area. The total area under the C,t curve, area$_T$, is 41.0 h mg/l for the 1000-mg dose. The i.v. value (Chapter 2, Section 4.3) found for a 250-mg dose is 21.3 h mg/l.

Bioavailability. Ampicillin has first-order disposition kinetics and so areas are proportional to doses and the bioavailability, F, may be calculated from equation (3.1).

$$F = 41.0/(4 \times 21.3) = 0.481$$

This value means that less than half of the oral dose reaches the plasma intact.

Apparent volume of distribution. The apparent volume of distribution estimated from the oral dose results is

$$V = F \times D/[k \times \text{area}_T(PO)]$$

$$V = 0.481 \times 1000/(0.418 \times 41.0) = 28.1 \text{ l}$$

This value is larger than that of 25.9 l from the i.v. study in Chapter 2 due to the effect of continuing absorption on the oral dose estimate of k. With drugs of short half-life it is preferable to estimate V from i.v. infusion data.

Renal clearance. The renal clearance from the oral dose may be assessed from the 3- to 4-h results in *Table 3.1*.

$$\text{mean excretion rate (3–4 h)} = 292.63 - 245.32 = 47.31 \text{ mg/h}$$

$$\text{mean plasma concentration} = (6.04 + 4.06)/2 = 5.05 \text{ mg/l}$$

$$Cl_r = 47.31/5.05 = 9.4 \text{ l/h}$$

Total clearance. For an oral dose the total clearance is the amount of drug reaching the plasma intact, divided by the total area under the C,t curve following the oral dose.

$$Cl_T = F \times D/\text{area}_T = 0.481 \times 1000/41.0 = 11.7 \text{ l/h}$$

Hepatic clearance. The difference between total and renal clearances gives an estimate of the hepatic clearance, Cl_h.

$$Cl_h = 11.7 - 9.4 = 2.3 \text{ l/h}$$

These values are similar to those for an i.v. dose of ampicillin (Chapter 2, Section 4.3).

Fraction absorbed. The fraction absorbed from the oral dose, F_a, is estimated from the results of the 24-h run set up below. The primary display is the table of results.

Summary of dialogue

```
CONTROL                        2 <E>      set run

SET RUN

   length of run h            24 <E>

   number of results           4 <E>

   times or interval           2 <E>      fixed interval

   enter interval              6 <E>

CONTROL                        5 <E>      start zero time

   primary display             1 <E>      table
```

At the end of the run:

```
                               <E>

CONTROL                       10 <E>      restart new drug
```

The program is then ready for the next run, which is with nortriptyline.

The results of this 24-h run are shown in *Table 3.2* taken from the results-log printed out at the end of the experiment. At 24 h there is an insignificant amount of drug left in the plasma and the outer distribution volume and so there is no need to continue the run for a further period.

The value of F_a is the sum of the values of X_m and X_u at complete elimination, divided by the dose.

$$F_a = (115.4 + 384.6)/1000 = 0.50$$

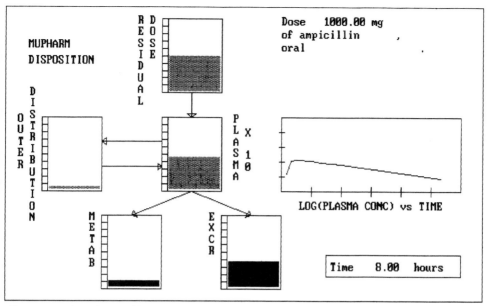

Press any key to continue

Figure 3.2 Ampicillin oral; 8-h disposition diagram.

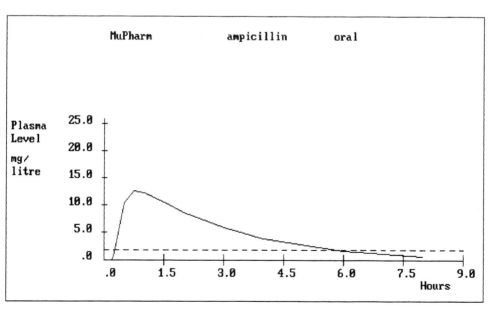

Press any key to continue

Figure 3.3 Ampicillin 1000 mg oral, area estimation.

Table 3.1 Ampicillin, area estimation.

```
**********MUPHARM RESULTS-LOG**********

Dose    1000.00 mg of ampicillin        oral

Numerical Details

time,h      cp,mg/l      xd,mg         xm,mg        xu,mg      response

  .25        1.44          .12           .29          .21         -
  .50       10.56         8.85          6.64        15.50         +
  .75       12.76        23.31         16.08        43.82         +
 1.00       12.50        36.37         25.64        73.93         +
 1.25       11.65        46.47         34.53       102.58         +
 1.50       10.69        53.70         42.63       129.04         +
 2.00        8.89        61.33         56.57       175.33         +
 3.00        6.04        60.08         77.09       245.32         +
 4.00        4.06        49.75         90.55       292.63         +
 6.00        1.78        27.60        105.05       345.20         -
 8.00         .76        13.40        111.13       368.00         -

AREA UNDER THE CURVE

The late time elimination constant is   .4182 1/h
The half life based on the last 3 points is    1.66 h
The extrapolation term is    1.82 hour.mg/litre
The estimate of total area is      41.03 hour.mg/litre
```

Hepatic extraction ratio. The hepatic extraction ratio is given by Chapter 1, equation (1.5):

$$E = 1 - F/F_a = 1 - 0.481/0.5 = 0.04$$

The first-pass effect is therefore small and the low bioavailability is mainly due to incomplete absorption. Ampicillin, a moderately strong acid, is relatively poorly absorbed in the gastro-intestinal tract. It is also transported in the bile to excretion in the faeces and these effects combine to give the low value of F_a.

Table 3.2 Ampicillin oral, estimation of fraction absorbed.

```
**********MUPHARM RESULTS-LOG**********

Dose    1000.00 mg of ampicillin        oral

Numerical Details

time,h      cp,mg/l      xd,mg         xm,mg        xu,mg      response

 6.00        1.78        27.60        105.05       345.20         -
12.00         .13         2.67        114.70       381.73         -
18.00         .01          .20        115.38       384.38         -
24.00         .00          .01        115.42       384.56         -
```

Ampicillin derivatives. The absorption of ampicillin from an oral dose is improved by using an ester of the acid, such as pivampicillin or talampicillin, both of which are rapidly hydrolysed after absorption, to give ampicillin.

An alternative to these esters is to use amoxycillin, a drug of chemical structure similar to that of ampicillin, which is almost completely absorbed from an oral dose; since it has antibiotic properties similar to those of ampicillin, it is generally preferred for oral administration. For i.v. administration, ampicillin is used because of its lower cost.

2.3.2 *Nortriptyline*

A short run for nortriptyline is set up exactly as for ampicillin except for the use of the different drug and the different dose of 50 mg. The primary display chosen is the disposition diagram, followed by a C,t plot. The dialogue following the restart different drug at the end of the last ampicillin run is as follows.

Summary of dialogue

DRUG	6 <E>	nortriptyline
CONTROL	1 <E>	prescribe drug
DOSE AND METHOD		
dose, mg	50 <E>	
multiple doses	<E>	
method of admin	3 <E>	oral
CONTROL	2 <E>	set run
SET RUN		
length of run h	3 <E>	
number of results	12 <E>	
times or interval	2 <E>	interval
enter interval h	0.25 <E>	
CONTROL	3 <E>	subject
SUBJECT		
1 standard, 2 own	1 <E>	

```
CONTROL                          5 <E>     start zero time

  primary display                3 <E>     disposition

                                           diagram

                                 <PrtSc>
```

At the end of the printout:

```
                                 <E>

CONTROL                          7 <E>     display

DISPLAY

  type                           1 <E>     C,t plot

                                 <PrtSc>
```

After the display has been printed:

```
                                 <E>

DISPLAY                          4 <E>     no more displays

CONTROL                          9 <E>     restart same drug
```

The program is then ready for the next run with nortriptyline.

The disposition diagram is shown in *Figure 3.4*. The top of the hatched area in the residual dose box indicates that the oral dose is almost completely absorbed. The plasma level is low and the outer disposition level is growing. Elimination is almost entirely by metabolism. An interesting result, in view of the relatively long half-life of nortriptyline, is that at 3 h the metabolism box contains more than half of the nortriptyline so far absorbed; this is due to the extensive first-pass metabolism of the drug. As is seen below, half the dose is metabolized before it reaches the main plasma volume.

The C,t results are shown in *Figure 3.5*.

Lag time. From the plot, the lag time is seen to be negligible.

C_{max}, t_{max}. The maximum point values are estimated as $C_{max} = 17$ μg/l, $t_{max} = 0.6$ h. The next oral run is for area estimation and is followed by a similar i.v. infusion run; in order to avoid transient toxic effects, the i.v. infusion dose is reduced to 10 mg over 0.5 h.

The details for both runs are set out in the following dialogue summary. Since they follow the first run with nortriptyline, drug, dose and subject need not be reselected for the oral run, but a new prescription is required for the i.v. infusion run.

Summary of dialogue

```
CONTROL                        2 <E>      set run

SET RUN

    length of run h            72 <E>

    number of results          17 <E>

    times or interval           1 <E>      specify times

    enter each time            0.25 <E> 0.5 <E> 0.75 <E>

                               1 <E>1.25 <E> 1.5 <E>

                               2 <E> 3 <E> 4 <E>

                               6 <E> 8<E> 12 <E>

                               24 <E> 36 <E> 48 <E>

                               60 <E> 72 <E>

CONTROL                         5 <E>      start zero time

    primary display             2 <E>      semilog plot
```

At the end of the run:

```
CONTROL                         8 <E>      area estimation

                               <E>

CONTROL                         9 <E>      restart same drug
```

The i.v. infusion run is then set up.

```
CONTROL                         1 <E>      prescribe drug

DOSE AND METHOD

    dose, mg                    10 <E>

    multiple doses             <E>        no

    method of admin             2 <E>      i.v. infusion
```

```
1st infusion time h          0.5 <E>

2nd infusion                 <E>        no

CONTROL                      5 <E>      start zero time

                             2 <E>      semilog plot
```

At the end of the run:

```
CONTROL                      8 <E>      area estimation

                             <E>

CONTROL                      9 <E>      restart same drug
```

Plots after these runs are not printed out. The program is left ready for the next run with nortriptyline.

The numerical results for the two runs are shown in *Tables 3.3* and *3.4*.

Half-life. The values of the elimination constant, k, for the two routes are 0.0224 h^{-1} for the oral route and 0.0238 h^{-1} for the i.v. infusion, giving plasma half-lives of 30.9 and 29.1 h. The small difference is due to continuing absorption in the later stages of the oral dose run, as found with ampicillin.

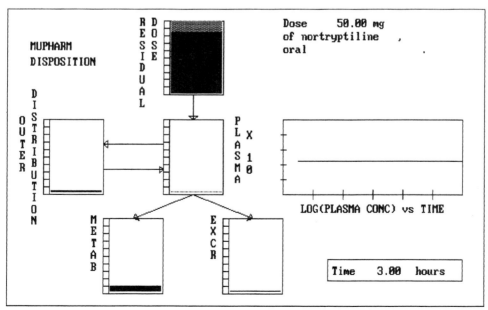

Press any key to continue

Figure 3.4 Nortriptyline oral, 3-h disposition.

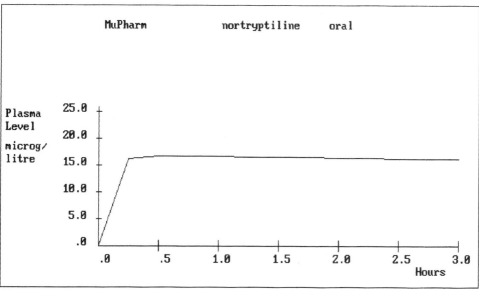

Press any key to continue

Figure 3.5 Nortriptyline 50 mg oral, short run.

Areas. The value of area$_T$(50 mg,oral) is 847 h μg/l or 0.847 h mg/l; area$_T$(10 mg,i.v.) is 336 h μg/l or 0.336 h mg/l.

Bioavailability. The bioavailability, F, is (from Chapter 1, equation 3.1):

$$F = \text{area}_T(50 \text{ mg,PO})/[5 \times \text{area}_T(10 \text{ mg,i.v.})] = 0.847/(5 \times 0.336) = 0.504$$

Apparent volume of distribution. The value of the volume of distribution V may be estimated directly from the i.v. results,

$$V = F \times D/[k \times \text{area}_T(10 \text{ mg,i.v.})] = 10/(0.0238 \times 0.336\} = 1251 \text{ l}$$

This very large value indicates that nortriptyline is widely distributed and is strongly bound outside the plasma. A feature of nortriptyline kinetics is that very little drug is present in the plasma; it is nearly all distributed to the outer volume of fluids and tissues.

Renal clearance. The renal clearance is estimated from the oral dose results in *Table 3.3* As there is little excretion of unchanged drug, an interval longer than that used with ampicillin is required to give a substantial change in X_u: the interval from 6 to 12 h is used.

The mean rate of urinary excretion of unchanged drug is:

$$\text{rate}(X)_u = (0.19 - 0.10)/6 = 0.015 \text{ mg/h}$$

The mean plasma concentration is:

$$C_{\text{mean}} = (15.53 + 13.97)/2 = 14.7 \text{ mg/l} = 0.0147 \text{ mg/l}$$

Table 3.3 Nortriptyline oral, area estimation.

```
**********MUPHARM RESULTS-LOG**********

Dose       50.00 mg of nortryptiline     oral

Numerical Details

time        cp,microg/l     xd,mg          xm,mg          xu,mg      response

   .25        16.36           .11            .32            .00          -
   .50        16.97           .29            .75            .01          -
   .75        16.92           .47           1.17            .01          -
  1.00        16.85           .64           1.60            .02          -
  1.25        16.78           .81           2.01            .02          -
  1.50        16.72           .98           2.43            .02          -
  2.00        16.59          1.31           3.24            .03          -
  3.00        16.32          1.92           4.82            .05          -
  4.00        16.06          2.49           6.34            .07          -
  6.00        15.53          3.51           9.20            .10          -
  8.00        15.00          4.37          11.85            .13          -
 12.00        13.97          5.69          16.56            .19          -
 24.00        11.11          7.42          27.10            .35          -
 36.00         8.69          7.31          33.91            .47          -
 48.00         6.71          6.44          38.43            .56          -
 60.00         5.14          5.36          41.49            .64          -
 72.00         3.92          4.31          43.61            .69          -

AREA UNDER THE CURVE

The late time elimination constant is    .0224 1/h
The half life based on the last 3 points is    30.95 h
The extrapolation term is    175.18 hour.microg/litre
The estimate of total area is       846.53 hour.microg/litre
```

Note the necessary conversion of the concentration units to match the rate units. The renal clearance is:

$$Cl_r = 0.015/0.0147 = 1.02 \text{ l/h}$$

This low value is mainly due to the high protein binding of nortriptyline (fraction bound = 0.95).

Total clearance. The total clearance estimated from the oral dose area is:

$$Cl_T = F \times D/\text{area}_T(50 \text{ mg,oral}) = 0.504 \times 50/0.847 = 29.8 \text{ l/h}$$

Hepatic clearance. The estimate of hepatic clearance is

$$Cl_h = Cl_T - Cl_r = 29.8 - 1.0 = 28.8 \text{ l/h}$$

The main clearance mechanism for nortriptyline is therefore metabolism.

Fraction absorbed. For the run to determine the fraction of the oral dose absorbed, F_a, the same dose of 50 mg is given and, since the last run was with the i.v. infusion, the prescription has to be re-entered. The run time is 144 h with results every 24 h. The table of results is chosen for the first presentation in order to check whether continuation of the run is necessary to secure complete elimination.

Table 3.4 Nortriptyline i.v., area estimation.

```
**********MUPHARM RESULTS-LOG**********

Dose      10.00 mg of nortryptiline    intravenous infusion
1st infusion    .50 h, 2nd infusion    .00 mg/h for    .00 h

Numerical Details
```

time	cp,microg/l	xd,mg	xm,mg	xu,mg	response
.25	274.35	2.37	1.59	.06	toxicity
.50	277.62	5.30	3.58	.13	toxicity
.75	5.61	5.84	4.00	.14	–
1.00	4.65	5.81	4.03	.14	–
1.25	4.62	5.77	4.06	.15	–
1.50	4.59	5.74	4.10	.15	–
2.00	4.54	5.67	4.16	.15	–
3.00	4.43	5.54	4.29	.15	–
4.00	4.33	5.41	4.42	.16	–
6.00	4.13	5.16	4.66	.17	–
8.00	3.93	4.92	4.89	.18	–
12.00	3.58	4.47	5.33	.19	–
24.00	2.69	3.36	6.40	.23	–
36.00	2.02	2.52	7.21	.26	–
48.00	1.52	1.90	7.82	.28	–
60.00	1.14	1.43	8.27	.30	–
72.00	.86	1.07	8.62	.31	–

```
AREA UNDER THE CURVE
The late time elimination constant is    .0238 1/h
The half life based on the last 3 points is    29.11 h
The extrapolation term is    36.01 hour.microg/litre
The estimate of total area is    336.01 hour.microg/litre
```

Summary of dialogue

```
CONTROL                         1 <E>    prescribe drug

DOSE AND METHOD

   dose, mg                     50 <E>

   multiple doses               <E>

   method of admin              3 <E>    oral

CONTROL                         2 <E>    set run

SET RUN

   length of run h              144 <E>

   number of results            6 <E>

   times or interval            2 <E>    interval
```

```
enter interval                24 <E>

CONTROL                        5 <E>    start zero time

  primary display              1 <E>    table
```

At 144 h it is seen from the upper part of *Table 3.5* that elimination is incomplete, as C_p and X_d are both significantly above zero; the run is therefore continued for another 144 h by using option 6 of the control menu.

```
                               <E>

CONTROL                        6 <E>    continue run

  repeat doses                 2 <E>    no
```

At the end of the continued run (lower part of *Table 3.5*), it is seen that the drug has been almost completely eliminated. Since this is the end of experiment 3, the program is stopped and the results-log is printed out.

```
                               <E>

CONTROL                       11 <E>    stop

Type your name

for labelling the printout     giles
```

The numerical results of the original run and its continuation are shown in *Table 3.5*. The fraction absorbed, F_a, is estimated by adding the totals shown in *Table 3.5*, of drug metabolized and excreted unchanged in the urine at 288 h, and dividing by the dose:

$$F_a = (49.11 + 0.86)/50 = 1.0$$

Nortriptyline is therefore completely absorbed from the oral dose.

Hepatic extraction ratio. The first pass effect estimated quantitatively by E is (from Chapter 1, equation 1.5):

$$E = 1 - F/F_a = 1 - 0.504/1.0 = 0.496$$

The low bioavailability of nortriptyline by the oral route is therefore due almost entirely to first-pass metabolism; half the dose is inactivated by metabolism before it reaches the main plasma volume.

2.4 Summary of experiment 3

Ampicillin and nortriptyline exhibit contrasting kinetic behaviour. When given by the oral route they both have bioavailabilities of around 0.5. With ampicillin the low value is due to incomplete absorption, whereas with nortriptyline it is due to a massive first-pass effect. Ampicillin is mainly cleared by urinary excretion of unchanged drug, while nortriptyline is cleared almost entirely by metabolism.

Table 3.5 Nortriptyline oral, fraction absorbed.

```
**********MUPHARM RESULTS-LOG**********

Dose      50.00 mg of nortryptiline      oral

Numerical Details

time       cp,microg/l    xd,mg          xm,mg           xu,mg        response
  24.00      11.11          7.42          27.10            .35          -
  48.00       6.71          6.44          38.43            .56          -
  72.00       3.92          4.31          43.61            .69          -
  96.00       2.25          2.64          46.17            .77          -
 120.00       1.29          1.55          47.51            .81          -
 144.00        .73           .90          48.23            .83          -


Continued run;
doses not repeated

Subject, standard 25y male, mass 70kg, height 183cm

Numerical Details

time       cp,microg/l    xd,mg          xm,mg           xu,mg        response
 168.00        .41           .51          48.63            .85          -
 192.00        .23           .29          48.85            .85          -
 216.00        .13           .16          48.98            .86          -
 240.00        .07           .09          49.05            .86          -
 264.00        .04           .05          49.08            .86          -
 288.00        .02           .03          49.11            .86          -
```

Ampicillin is rapidly eliminated and the estimate of the late time elimination rate constant following oral dose is affected by continuing absorption from the oral dose

Nortriptyline has a very large apparent volume of distribution, indicating that it is strongly bound outside the plasma.

3. PHARMACOKINETIC PARAMETERS FOLLOWING INTRAMUSCULAR DOSE

Lag time, slow and incomplete absorption may occur after an i.m. dose, but because the absorbed drug enters directly into the main plasma volume rather than via the hepatic portal vein, there is no first pass effect. Apparent incomplete absorption may in some cases be due to very slow uptake in the final stages of a study, so that the resulting plasma and urine concentrations are below the limit of analytical detection.

The pharmacokinetic parameters relevant to the i.m. route, in addition to those for the i.v. route are t_{lag}, C_{max}, t_{max} and F.

4. EXPERIMENT 4: TO DETERMINE KINETIC PARAMETERS RESULTING FROM AN INTRAMUSCULAR DOSE OF GENTAMICIN

Gentamicin is an antibiotic which is normally given by the i.v. and i.m. routes, because it is poorly absorbed from the gastro-intestinal tract.

4.1 Objectives

The objective of this study is to determine pharmacokinetic parameters for gentamicin given by i.m. injection to the standard subject.

4.2 Experimental plan

A suitable i.m. dose for gentamicin is 120 mg. A first short run is required to determine t_{lag}, C_{max} and t_{max}. As in experiment 3, a run of 3 h with results every 0.25 h is made. The primary display is the disposition diagram and a C,t plot of results is generated at the end of the run.

Since the half-life of gentamicin is around 2.5 h (Appendix II), the second run, for estimating area, is set for 12 h; results are taken at the same timings as for ampicillin (Chapter 2, Section 4.2) with the addition of a 12-h result. A third run to estimate the i.v. area is made and, since gentamicin is a toxic drug, the dose is reduced to an i.v. infusion of 30 mg over 0.5 h.

There is no need for a run for calculating the fraction absorbed since as there is no first-pass effect with an i.m. dose, the fraction absorbed, F_a, is equal to the bioavailability, F.

4.3 Runs and results

The three runs are set up to follow consecutively, with the following dialogue:

Summary of dialogue

```
DRUG                         12 <E>    gentamicin

CONTROL                       1 <E>    prescribe drug

DOSE AND METHOD

   dose, mg                 120 <E>

   multiple doses               <E>    no

   method of admin            5 <E>    i.m.

CONTROL                        2 <E>    set run

SET RUN

   length of run h            3 <E>

   number of results         12 <E>

   times or interval          2 <E>    interval

   enter times interval     0.25 <E>
```

```
CONTROL                          3 <E>      subject

SUBJECT

  1 standard, 2 own              1 <E>

CONTROL                          5 <E>      start zero time

  primary display               3 <E>      disposition

                                            diagram

                                 <PrtSc>
```

At the end of the print-out:

```
                                 <E>

CONTROL                          7 <E>      display

DISPLAY

  type                           1 <E>      C,t plot

                                 <PrtSc>
```

After the display has been printed:

```
                                 <E>

DISPLAY                          4 <E>      no more displays

CONTROL                          9 <E>      restart same drug
```

The program is then ready for the i.m. area estimation; the only change required for this run is in the timing of results.

```
CONTROL                          2 <E>      set run

SET RUN

  length of run h               12 <E>

  number of results             12 <E>

  times or interval             1 <E>      specify times

  enter each time               0.25 <E> 0.5 <E> 0.75 <E>
```

```
                                      1 <E>1.25 <E> 1.5 <E>

                                      2 <E> 3 <E> 4 <E>

                                      6 <E> 8 <E> 12 <E>
CONTROL                               5 <E>      start zero time

  primary display                     2 <E>      semilog plot
```
At the end of the run:
```
                                      <E>

CONTROL                               8 <E>      area estimate

                                      <E>

CONTROL                               9 <E>      restart same drug
```
A third run, for estimating the i.v. area is then set up. The prescription needs to be changed to 30 mg over 0.5 h, i.v. infusion; the run timings are the same.
```
CONTROL                               1 <E>      prescribe drug

DOSE AND METHOD

  dose, mg                            30 <E>

  multiple doses                      <E>        no

  method of admin                     2 <E>      i.v. infusion

    infusion time                     0.5 <E>

    second infusion                   <E>        no

CONTROL                               5 <E>      start zero time

  primary display                     2 <E>      semilog graph
```
At the end of the run:
```
                                      <E>

CONTROL                               8 <E>      area estimate

                                      <E>
```

```
CONTROL                                 11 <E>   stop

Type your name

for labelling the printout              giles
```

The results-log may then be printed.

Disposition diagram. The disposition diagram is shown in *Figure 3.6*. The residual dose box is empty at 3 h but as shown by the stippled area, it has been filled to the top, indicating that all the i.m. dose has been taken up into the plasma. Elimination is entirely by urinary excretion of unchanged drug; there is no metabolism.

The results for the short run are shown in *Figure 3.7*.

Absorption parameters. t_{lag} = 0.15 h; C_{max} = 7.0 mg/l; t_{max} = 0.5 h.

The results for the i.m. area estimation run are shown in *Table 3.6*.

Plasma half-life. The value of the elimination constant is 0.287 h^{-1} by both routes; the plasma half-life is 2.42 h.

Area. $area_T$ (120 mg,i.m.), 27.9; $area_T$ (30 mg,i.v.), 7.04 h mg/l.

Bioavailability. The value of F is:

$$F = 27.9/(4 \times 7.04) = 0.99$$

For the i.m. route, $F_a = F$. The value of 0.99 for F means that effectively the entire i.m. dose is taken up into the plasma.

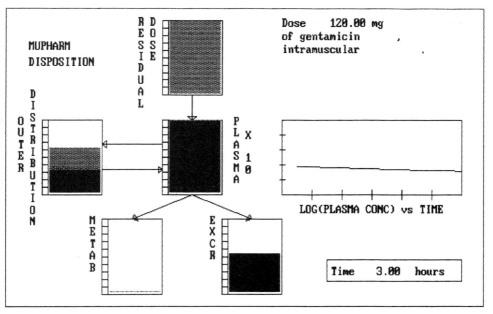

Press any key to continue

Figure 3.6 Gentamicin i.m., disposition diagram.

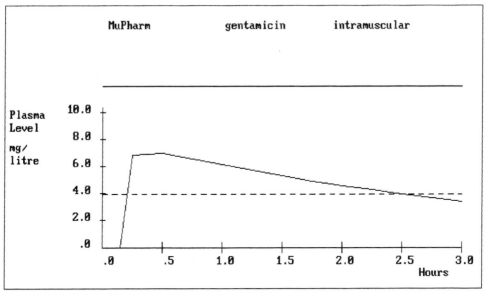

Press any key to continue

Figure 3.7 Gentamicin 120 mg i.m., short run.

Table 3.6 Gentamicin i.m., area estimation.

```
**********MUPHARM RESULTS-LOG**********

Dose      120.00 mg of gentamicin      intramuscular

Numerical Details
```

time,h	cp,mg/l	xd,mg	xm,mg	xu,mg	response
.25	6.90	33.74	.00	2.11	+
.50	7.03	73.24	.00	9.77	+
.75	6.63	75.04	.00	17.18	+
1.00	6.19	70.97	.00	24.12	+
1.25	5.76	66.24	.00	30.59	+
1.50	5.36	61.68	.00	36.61	+
2.00	4.64	53.45	.00	47.43	+
3.00	3.49	40.12	.00	64.93	−
4.00	2.62	30.11	.00	78.06	−
6.00	1.47	16.97	.00	95.32	−
8.00	.83	9.56	.00	105.05	−
12.00	.26	3.04	.00	113.62	−

```
AREA UNDER THE CURVE

The late time elimination constant is   .2868 1/h
The half life based on the last 3 points is   2.42 h
The extrapolation term is      .92 hour.mg/litre
The estimate of total area is      27.92 hour.mg/litre
```

Volume of distribution. The volume of distribution is given by Chapter 1, equation (1.9) as

$$V = F \times D/[k \times \text{area}_T(D,\text{i.m.})] = 0.99 \times 120/(0.287 \times 27.9) = 14.8 \text{ l}$$

This low value indicates that gentamicin is not widely distributed.

Renal clearance. From the data in *Table 3.6*, the 3- to 4-h renal clearance of gentamicin following i.m. dose is

$$\text{rate}(X)_u = 78.06 - 64.93 = 13.1 \text{ mg/h}$$

$$C_{\text{mean}} = (3.49 + 2.62)/2 = 3.06 \text{ mg/l}$$

$$Cl_r = 13.1/3.06 = 4.28 \text{ l/h}$$

Total clearance. The total clearance is

$$Cl_T = F \times D/\text{area}_T(D,\text{i.m.}) = 0.99 \times 120/27.9 = 4.26 \text{ l/h}$$

Hepatic clearance. The above two clearances are the same within the likely estimation error and so the hepatic clearance is negligible. This result is also seen from *Table 3.6*, where X_m remains zero throughout the run. Clearance of gentamicin is entirely by urinary excretion of unchanged drug.

4.4 Conclusions from experiment 4

Gentamicin is well absorbed from an i.m. dose and has only a limited distribution outside the plasma. It is not metabolized and is excreted entirely as unchanged drug.

5. PROBLEMS

1. Determine pharmacokinetic parameters for oxprenolol (properties, Appendix II) following an oral dose of 80 mg to the standard subject. Use the results from question 2, Chapter 2, for the assessment of bioavailability.

2. Determine the pharmacokinetic parameters of the antibiotic amoxycillin, given by the oral route, with an additional i.v. infusion run to determine i.v. area. Amoxycillin is available on an extra drug file (Chapter 4 and Appendix VI). Compare the kinetic parameters with those for ampicillin.

3. Make runs to determine pharmacokinetic parameters for phenobarbitone following an i.m. dose of 300 mg.

Operational Details for the Simulation Model

1. GENERAL CONSIDERATIONS

The single-dose experiments in Chapters 2 and 3 have shown you how to use some of the main features of the MuPharm simulation. It is now time to look at the full range of the program, both in terms of the structure of the model and the operational aspects for its use.

When the MuPharm program has been loaded and the title pages have been passed (by pressing <ENTER>, denoted here as previously by <E>), you first see the DRUG SELECTION menu. The choice of drug is made by number (Section 2) and the CONTROL menu then appears. This menu offers 11 different options for further development of the run. These options and what follows from them are outlined in Section 3.

At any point in the dialogue, explanatory 'help' is made available on typing 'q' in answer to any of the dialogue requests.

Numerical responses to questions are restricted to lie within certain ranges. If a reply is outside the designated range the message

```
It has to be between ... and ... Try again
```

appears. A number within this range should then be entered.

The screen is cleared of dialogue when the final requested information has been entered at the keyboard, followed by <E>. When the screen contains displays such as tables or graphs of results without any requirement for further information, the message

```
Press any key to continue
```

appears and the screen display persists until this instruction is obeyed.

In the following summary, as above and in previous chapters, the dialogue and associated information are printed in a different typeface to the text.

2. DRUG SELECTION

The drug selection menu presented on the screen is as follows:

```
DRUG SELECTION

   1. Ampicillin          11. Temazepam
```

```
 2.  Aspirin            12.  Gentamicin

 3.  Digitoxin          13.  Digoxin

 4.  Indomethacin       14.  Theophylline

 5.  Kanamycin          15.  Lignocaine

 6.  Nortriptyline      16.  Carbamazepine

 7.  Oxprenolol         17.  Benzpenicillin

 8.  Paracetamol        18.  Thiopentone

 9.  Phenobarbitone     19.  Atenolol

10.  Phenytoin          20.  Diamorphine
```

```
Enter a number for the drug; enter q for a list of uses;
press <ENTER> alone to specify use of an extra drug file
```

When 'q' is entered in reply to DRUG SELECTION, a list of the purposes for which the drugs are used in the simulation is presented on the screen (see Chapter 2, Section 2.2, Table 2.1).

The arrangement for extra drug files may be used to add to the 20 drugs on the main file. An extra drug, amoxycillin, is supplied with the program to show how the scheme works. The file name is AMOXYCIL. Information on setting up your own drug files is given in Appendix VI.

When <ENTER> alone is pressed, the user is asked:

```
Enter name of file containing drug factors

(* to return to DRUG SELECTION menu)
```

The escape route is provided in case the option was selected by mistake.

3. THE CONTROL MENU

After selecting a drug, the main CONTROL menu is displayed, with 11 choices as follows:

```
CONTROL

  1.  Prescribe drug          < —

  2.  Set timings for run     < —
```

```
 3. Specify subject         < —

 4. Change factors

 5. Start run at zero time

 6. Continue run

 7. Display results

 8. Estimate area under C,t plot

 9. Restart, same drug

10. Restart, different drug

11. Stop
```

You must complete the first three options, which are initially marked, in order to start a new run, otherwise an error message is displayed:

```
Prescription, run or subject details incomplete
```

As each of the first three options is completed, the associated marker disappears.

Option 4 may then be chosen if changes are required to the present drug or subject factors or to the precision or speed of the calculations, or to the lag time; otherwise you proceed to option 5 to start the calculations.

The remaining options are for use after the end of a run. If you wish to continue the run for a further period, option 6 is used. Option 7 branches to the DISPLAY sub-menu with choices for the display of results stored at this point. Option 8 gives the AREA calculation leading to the presentation on the screen of values of the late time elimination constant, the plasma half-life and the area under the C,t curve. Options 9 and 10 are used preparatory to setting up new runs.

Option 11 takes you out of the program and enables you to print out the results-log, which gives tables of all the numerical results obtained during the session, together with the prescriptions used and any changes made in factors through the CHANGE menu.

The dialogue for finishing a session is:

```
CONTROL 11                <E>      stop

Type your name

for labelling the printout    giles
```

To display or print the results-log requires a command which depends on the machine in use and is described in the implementation notes which accompany the program.

The options arising from the CONTROL menu and the dialogue associated with them are considered in detail in the following sections.

3.1 **Prescribe drug**

The sequence of operations required to prescribe the chosen drug is structured with prompted input as follows.

```
DOSE AND METHOD OF ADMINISTRATION
```

```
For repeated doses this is the maintenance dose; a
loading dose if required, is entered later. For IV
infusion this is the total dose for the first, if there
is a second infusion it is entered later
```

At the bottom of the screen, in a standard position used for all the prompts requiring the user to enter a response, there appears:

```
Enter the dose of <drug name> in mg
```

The appropriate figure followed by <E> is entered. The next prompt is:

```
Multiple doses, enter the repeated dose interval in h,
press <ENTER> only for no repetition
```

If you select multiple doses, you are then asked to:

```
Enter the total number of doses
```

The next section of dialogue is concerned with the method of administration.

```
Method of administration
```

```
1. IV bolus
```

```
2. IV infusion
```

```
3. Oral
```

```
4. Oral sustained release
```

```
5. IM
```

```
Choose the method required by number
```

This then leads on to a different set of questions according to the method chosen, returning on completion to the CONTROL menu.

```
1. IV bolus
```

No further information is required here unless the dose is to be repeated, when the following appears.

```
If required enter in mg a loading dose greater than the
dose; if not press <ENTER> alone
```

```
2. IV infusion
```

```
Enter the duration of the first infusion in h
```

If there is to be only one infusion, this is the duration of infusion of the total dose already entered. If a second infusion is to follow, this sets up the duration for the first infusion.

```
For a second infusion, enter the rate in mg/h; if none
required press <ENTER> alone
```

If you enter a non-zero number here the duration of the second infusion is requested.

```
Enter the duration of the second infusion in hours
following the end of the first infusion
```

A complication can arise if the two infusions are to be repeated, the dose interval should then be longer than the sum of the two infusion periods. If it is not, a message appears and an opportunity is given to increase the dose interval.

```
The dose interval is too short, it should be at least
equal to the sum of the infusion times
```

```
Enter a greater value for the dose interval
```

```
3. Oral
```

With some drugs on the main list a message

```
The oral route is not available for this drug
```

appears. Drugs for which this message is displayed are: kanamycin and gentamicin (very poor absorption from the GIT); lignocaine and diamorphine (extensive first-pass metabolism); and benzylpenicillin (the drug is almost completely inactivated in the acid environment of the stomach).

On pressing <E> after this message, you are returned to the CONTROL menu, whereupon another prescription may be entered.

There are no further requests for information for the oral route in the prescription dialogue, unless the dose is to be repeated. If it is you will be asked:

```
Enter if required a loading dose larger than the main
dose; if not required press <ENTER> alone
```

A non-zero answer leads to the further request:

```
For a single loading dose enter 1; for a divided loading
dose enter 2
```

If 2 is entered then:

```
How many divided doses are required?
```

then:

```
Enter the interval in hours between them
```

A limitation imposed is that the loading dose should be completed within the first main dose interval. If this is found not to be the case, a message appears:

```
The loading dose should be completed within the first
main dose interval
```

You should then re-enter details of the divided loading dose.

```
4. Oral sustained release (see chapter 6)
```

For the drugs which are not available by the oral route, the message described under 3 appears. The dialogue here sets up the details for the dosage form. The dose entered should be the effective oral dose (see Chapter 6, Section 2). The lag time is specified later, under the factor change option (4) of the CONTROL menu.

The dialogue for setting up the sustained release dosage form (see Chapter 6, Sections 2 and 3 for further information) is:

```
Enter the first release period in h
```

then:

```
If required, enter second release period in h following
the first, press <ENTER> alone for no second period.
```

If there is a second period:

```
Enter as a decimal, the fraction of the dose released in
the first period
```

A final option offers the possibility of giving a rapid release loading dose at the same time as the sustained release preparation:

```
If required enter a rapid release loading dose in mg; if
not press <ENTER> alone
```

A limitation for repeated sustained release doses is that the repeated dose interval should be longer than the first release period and also longer than half the sum of the two release periods. If these conditions are not met a message appears and you are invited to specify a longer dosing interval.

```
The repeated dose interval should be greater than the 1st
period and than half the sum of the two periods
```

```
Enter a longer dosing interval
```

5. IM

With some of the drugs a message

```
The IM route is not available for this drug
```

appears; you are then returned to the CONTROL menu.

If repeated doses have been prescribed, the possibility of a loading dose is offered:

```
If required enter in mg a loading dose greater than the
dose; if not press <ENTER> alone
```

3.2 Set timings for the run

This option is chosen next from the CONTROL menu. The dialogue is as follows.

```
SET UP THE RUN

The run should be planned in advance so that the length,
the number of results and the timings of results may be
entered in reply to the dialogue requests
```

```
Enter the length of the run in h
```

Then:

```
Enter the number of times that results are required
```

You should have worked out this number in the plan for the experiment.

```
To specify each time for a result enter 1;
```

```
for a fixed interval between results, enter 2
```

When the answer is '1', the times are entered successively, each followed by <E>.

```
Enter each time in h; press <ENTER> after each time
```

When the answer is '2', you give the time interval between results:

```
Enter the time interval in hours
```

Times at which results are required should not exceed the maximum time expressed by the run length. If they do a message is displayed:

```
Output time exceeds the run length, try again
```

and you are then repositioned in the dialogue to repeat the setting of the run.

The arrangements for setting the run are then complete and you are returned to the CONTROL menu.

3.3 Specify subject

This option permits you to select the standard subject or a subject which you define in terms of age, body mass, height and sex, or a preset subject whose characteristics have been set up in an extra subject file.

Information on setting up your own extra subject files is given in Appendix VII. An extra subject file is supplied with the program, it has the file name SUBJ3HD, and is a 50-year-old female of height 155 cm and body mass 75 kg with a 40% loss of hepatic function.

The dialogue for selecting the subject is as follows.

```
SET UP THE SUBJECT

The standard subject is a 25y old male, bodymass 70kg,
height 183cm. To set up your own subject, sex, age, mass
and height are entered. Subject factors are then modified
in the program to comply with these values. Subject
factors may be further modified through the CHANGE menu.


Type 1 for the standard subject, 2 to define your own

Press <ENTER> alone to load an extra subject file
```

On response 1, the user is returned to the CONTROL menu with the standard subject factor values set.

On response 2, the sequence of dialogue to define the subject appears as follows:

```
Enter the height in cm, 1 foot = 30.5 cm

Enter the body mass in kg, 1 stone = 6.35 kg

Enter the age in years

Enter 1 for male, 2 for female
```

If <ENTER> alone is pressed, you are asked to:

```
Enter name of the file containing subject details

(* to return to SUBJECT menu)
```

On completion of this option, you have supplied all the necessary information for starting a run. You are returned to the CONTROL menu, where you have a choice of options 4 and 5 (also 6 if a run has been completed and is to be continued).

3.4 Change factors

This option can only be entered once options 1, 2 and 3 — the obligatory requirements for a run — have been completed. The CHANGE sub-menu appears which enables you to change factors relating to the calculation, the drug, the subject and the lag time.

```
CHANGE FACTORS

1 alter the iteration time

2 change drug factor(s)

3 change subject factor(s)

4 change lag time

5 no further changes
```

The changes made are temporary and the factors revert to their standard values on reloading.

When option 9 of the CONTROL menu, `restart same drug` is chosen, all changes are maintained; with option 10, `restart different drug` changes to iteration time and to subject factors are maintained, but changes to drug factors and to lag time are lost.

```
1. Alter the iteration time
```

The program solves the mathematical equations defining the model at discrete time steps, the increment between steps being the iteration time interval.

The option to change the iteration interval from its normal value of 0.01 h may be used to speed up or slow down the calculations. A value above 0.02 h may lead to numerical inaccuracy and to instability of the solution. The effects of altering the iteration interval are discussed in Appendix VIII.

A reduction of the iteration interval may be used to slow down the changes in the disposition diagram so that they can be more easily followed (Chapter 2, Section 4.3); a change to 0.001 h is suggested.

The dialogue for changing the iteration interval is:

```
CHANGE ITERATION TIME INTERVAL

The standard interval is 0.01 h. Increasing the interval
speeds up the calculations but reduces the precision.
Reducing it has the opposite effects. The iteration
interval should not be greater than 0.02h.


The present value is <interval> enter the new value
```

where <interval> implies display of the current value.

2. Change drug factors

This option first lists 19 numbered factors, one of which is not used, and 16 of which are changeable in the dialogue. These factors are discussed in Appendix IV and are not considered in detail here.
The dialogue for change is:

```
Enter factor number, press <ENTER> alone to complete
```

After entering a number:

```
The present value of drug factor <number> is <value>

Enter the new value
```

After setting the value, further factors may be changed; or if <ENTER> alone is pressed, you are returned to the CHANGE sub-menu.

3. Change subject factors

The SUBJECT FACTOR sub-menu lists nine numbered factors, eight of which are changeable in the dialogue. These factors are discussed in detail in Appendix III.
The dialogue for change is:

```
Enter factor number, press <ENTER> alone to complete
```

<ENTER> alone returns you to the CHANGE sub-menu.
On entering a valid factor number, the new value is requested:

```
The present value of subject factor <number> is <value>

Enter the new value
```

You are returned to allow a further subject factor to be changed; alternatively pressing <ENTER> alone here returns you to the CHANGE sub-menu.

4. Change lag time

On selecting this option, which is only available for oral and i.m. routes, the following dialogue ensues:

```
LAG TIME

Lag time applies to oral and IM routes. For compressed
tablets and capsules, it is likely to be in the range 0.1
to 0.5h; for sustained release preparations, it is
usually longer, around 1h
```

```
The present lag time is <time>; enter the new value in h
```

```
5. No further changes
```

After completing a change, you are returned to the CHANGE sub-menu; when the required changes are completed, you choose option 5 to return to the main CONTROL menu.

3.5 Start run at zero time

This option in the CONTROL menu is used to start the run at zero time. First a primary display has to be selected. The choice of primary display is between a table of numerical results, a five-cycle semilog plot of plasma concentration and a diagram showing the disposition of the drug. After entering option 5, the following prompt appears:

```
Do you want the primary display to be
```

```
1) tabular, 2) graphical, 3) disposition diagram, 4)
slowed version of 3?
```

On pressing <ENTER> after this choice has been made, the calculations begin and the display appears and grows as the results are calculated.

Option 4 is useful for short runs so that the changes in the disposition diagram may be followed easily. The iteration time is reduced by a factor of 10 and is restored to the previous value when the diagram is completed.

At the end of the run when the display is complete, the following message appears:

```
Press any key to continue
```

The primary display persists until any key is pressed; you are then returned to the CONTROL menu.

If the subject is unfortunate enough to die of an overdose during a run, the primary display stops and a message appears.

```
Your subject has died of an overdose; reset subject and
prescription
```

In this case, on pressing <E> you are returned to the CONTROL menu, where options 1 and 3 are arrowed, indicating the need to chose a new subject and represcribe the drug.

3.6. Continue run

This option continues the existing run for another equal period from the end of the previous run. First you are asked whether you wish to

```
Repeat doses in continued run? 1 yes, 2 no
```

Reply 1 is used when the run is to be continued in order to reach a steady state with repeated doses; reply 2 is used when the continuation is to secure complete elimination of the drug, as in urinary excretion studies.

When reply 2 is chosen, the doses are cancelled completely and so for a new run starting at zero time, the drug must be re-prescribed.

Between the original run and a continuation, a new prescription may be entered and drug and subject factors may be changed. Since the continued run is based on the same framework of iteration interval and timing of results as the original run, result timings, iteration interval and lag time cannot be changed.

The CONTINUE option is useful for setting up long runs in which each time for a result has to be entered. For example, for a peak and trough, repeated dose run of 576 h, a run of 144 h is first set up and the timings entered. At the end of this run, if the results are satisfactory, it is continued with doses three times to give the total time of 576 h. In the continued runs the peak and trough timings are automatically entered.

The primary display for a continued run follows on from that for the original one. At the end of the continuation, the display persists until <ENTER> is pressed; you are then returned to the CONTROL menu.

3.7 Display results

Choice of this option leads to the appearance of the DISPLAY sub-menu.

```
DISPLAY OPTIONS

1. Plasma concentration/time curve

2. Semilog plot of plasma concentration

3. Display current prescription and subject

4. No more displays
```

The first option gives a simple plot of plasma concentration against time, the scales on the axes are adjusted automatically for the data.

The second option gives a logarithmic axis for the concentration values, further dialogue enables you to control the scale of this vertical axis.

```
Type minimum concentration to be displayed on axis. Press
<ENTER> alone for automatic scaling
```

```
Type number of log cycles in display. Press <ENTER> alone
for automatic choice
```

This dialogue enables you to scale the graph according to information obtained from the primary graphical display. Alternatively, by responding with <ENTER> alone, the scaling is made automatically, according to the data.

The third option, Display current prescription and subject is used, if required, for graphical displays as the details of prescription and route are not shown on the graphs. This information, together with details of any parameter changes, may always be obtained from the results-log, which can be printed out at the end of each session.

The fourth option returns you to the CONTROL menu.

3.8 Estimate area under *C,t* plot

This option is not available for results from an i.v. bolus prescription. If it is selected after such a run, a message appears:

```
The area calculation is unsuitable for IV bolus

use IV infusion
```

You are then returned to the CONTROL menu.

For results from other methods of administration, the choice of this option results in the following display:

```
AREA UNDER THE CURVE

The late time elimination constant is <k>

The half life based on the last 3 points is <t₁/₂>
```

The half life based on the last 3 points is $<t_{1/2}>$

```
The extrapolation term is <areaₑ>
```

The extrapolation term is $<area_e>$

```
The estimate of total area is <areaᴛ>
```

The estimate of total area is $<area_T>$

```
The elimination constant is determined by a regression
analysis on the last three values of ln(C) and t
```

If the last concentration in the set of results is less than 0.01 in whichever of the concentration units are being used, the calculation of the elimination constant, k, may be unreliable. In this case, it is considered that the run has been continued long enough to make the extrapolated area negligible. Values of k and half-life are not calculated and the area given is the sum of the trapezium areas.

The display when this result occurs is:

```
AREA UNDER THE CURVE

The last C value is too small to estimate k;

the extrapolated area has been set to zero;

for an estimate of half life use a shorter run.
```

```
The extrapolation term is zero
```

The estimate of total area is $<area_T>$

On pressing <ENTER>, the screen display is replaced by the CONTROL menu.

3.9 Restart, same drug

This choice from the CONTROL menu bypasses the choice of drug and retains the details of prescription, run and subject as well as any factor changes which have been made. The CONTROL menu reappears, from which any required changes for a second run with the same drug may be made.

3.10 Restart, different drug

This option takes you right back to DRUG SELECTION. After the new drug has been chosen a new prescription is required but run and subject details are retained unless altered through the CONTROL menu.

3.11 Stop

The stop option ends a MuPharm session. A message appears:

```
Type your name for labelling print-out
```

After entering a name, execution returns to the operating system prompt.

As described in the implementation notes, at this stage the results-log, containing details of the numerical results, the prescriptions, the subjects used and any factor changes made during the session may be displayed on the screen or printed out.

CHAPTER 5

Continuous and Multiple Dosing Regimens, Intravenous and Oral Doses. Studies with Lignocaine, Ampicillin and Carbamazepine

1. INTRODUCTION

The target for continuous and repeated dosing schemes is to maintain plasma concentrations of a drug above the minimum active level and safely below the minimum toxic level.

Continuous dosing is effected by a prolonged, constant rate, i.v. infusion. The plasma concentration, C, of the drug rises as the infusion proceeds, until a steady state is reached at which the rate of elimination, which is proportional to C for first-order elimination, becomes equal to the rate of infusion. The curve flattens to a constant concentration plateau, as shown in *Figure 5.1*.

The plateau concentration is the steady-state plasma level. The infusion rate required to give a target steady-state plasma level of a drug may be calculated by considering the rate of elimination.

If C_{SS} is the target level required, then the rate of elimination at this concentration is $Cl_T \times C_{SS}$ in mg/h, where Cl_T is the total clearance of the drug (Chapter 1, Section 10.3); therefore if rate$(X)_e$ is the rate of elimination in mg/h

$$\text{rate}(X)_e = Cl_T \times C_{SS}$$

At the steady state, the constant infusion rate, rate$(X)_i$, in mg/h is equal to the elimination rate, rate$(X)_i$ = rate$(X)_e$, i.e.

$$\text{rate}(X)_i = Cl_T \times C_{SS}$$

$$(5.1)$$

Cl_T may be calculated from the area under the C,t curve, determined from a single-dose experiment with the drug. By choosing C_{SS} as a suitable plasma concentration above the minimum active level but below the toxic level (see Appendix II for values of these levels for the different drugs), an infusion regimen may be set up. Target levels of 2–4 times the minimum active level are suitable for many regimens.

In experiment 5 below, an infusion schedule is developed for lignocaine, a drug which is rapidly eliminated.

2. EXPERIMENT 5: INTRAVENOUS INFUSION REGIMEN FOR LIGNOCAINE

2.1 Objective

The objective is to develop an i.v. infusion regimen with lignocaine which will give a rapid attainment of active plasma levels of the drug, followed by a constant plasma concentration of lignocaine which is well into the active range and safely below the toxic level.

2.2 Plan

Lignocaine is used for the treatment of arrhythmias; it is very rapidly metabolized in the liver resulting in a large first-pass effect when given orally and has a short half-life of around 1.5 h. Because of the first-pass effect the oral route is not used for systemic treatment and the drug is usually given by the i.v. route. As a result of the rapid metabolism, relatively large infusion rates are required.

From Appendix II it is seen that the minimum active plasma level is 2 mg/l while the toxic level is 6 mg/l, the therapeutic index C_{tox}/C_{act} of 3.0 is relatively low. A target steady-state plasma concentration, C_{SS}, is set at 4 mg/l.

The first run is to estimate the total clearance of lignocaine. From Appendix II, the half-life is 1.5 h, a run of 6 h is therefore sufficient for determining the area under the C,t curve. An i.v. infusion of 200 mg over 0.5 h is given.

The value of the area under the C,t curve is used to estimate the total clearance and hence the required infusion rate to give the target value for C_{SS}, using equation (5.1).

In the dialogue, a first infusion is given as a total dose over a given period. To set up a run to test the calculated infusion rate, a 12-h run is set up with a total dose of $(12 \times rate(X)_i)$ mg of lignocaine given as an i.v. infusion over 12 h. In order to see the magnitudes of plasma concentrations clearly (this can sometimes be awkward with a semilog graph), a C,t plot is chosen to display the results.

In the treatment of arrythmias it is necessary to reach the active level as quickly as possible. This result is achieved by giving an i.v. bolus dose or a short infusion, to take the plasma level rapidly to the active level; the maintenance dose then continues as a second infusion.

Two further runs are made with the same maintenance dose and short loading dose infusions of 100 mg/0.02 h and 200 mg/0.05 h. A C,t graph is printed out for the 100-mg/ 6-h run. For the 200-mg run only the early results are of concern and so a run of 1 h with results every 0.1 h is made.

2.3 Runs and results

The details of the area estimation run are set out below. It is assumed that you are now familiar with the dialogue and so the run details are given simply as the information necessary for you to set up the run. These details are listed in the right order for entering into the program. Any problems with the dialogue should be resolved by reference to Chapter 4.

The first run, for area estimation, is set up as follows.

```
Run details
```

```
Lignocaine, 200mg IV infusion over 0.5h;
```

```
run length 6h, 10 results at 0.25, 0.5, 0.75, 1, 1.25,
1.5, 2, 3, 4, 6h;
```

```
standard subject;
```

```
run, primary display, table;
```

```
area estimate;
```

```
restart same drug.
```

Results for this run are shown in *Table 5.1*; values from the area estimation are:

$$k = 0.448 \text{ h}^{-1}, \quad t_{1/2} = 1.55 \text{ h}, \quad \text{area}_T = 4.53 \text{ h mg/l}$$

The total clearance is calculated using equation (1.12) (Chapter 1, Section 10.3). D is 200 mg and F is 1.0 for the i.v. route.

$$Cl_T = F \times D/\text{area}_T = 200/4.53 = 44.2 \text{ l/h}$$

The required rate of infusion of lignocaine in mg/h at the target plasma level of 4 mg/ l is now estimated using equation (5.1):

$$\text{rate}(X)_i = 44.2 \times 4 = 176.8 \text{ mg/h}$$

The above figure is rounded to 175 mg/h (2.9 mg/min).

The next run is to test this infusion schedule: the run length is 12 h and results are obtained every 0.5 h. The total dose is $175 \times 12 = 2100$ mg i.v. infusion over 12 h. Since this run follows the previous one after restarting with the same drug, a new dose and new run times are required but there is no need to respecify the subject.

```
Run details
```

```
Lignocaine 2100mg IV infusion over 12h;
```

```
run length 12h, 24 results at 0.5h intervals;
```

```
start, primary display, graph;
```

```
display and print C,t plot;
```

```
restart same drug
```

Table 5.1 Lignocaine i.v., area estimation.

```
**********MUPHARM RESULTS-LOG**********

Dose      200.00 mg of lignocaine       intravenous infusion
1st infusion      .50 h, 2nd infusion    .00 mg/h for     .00 h

Numerical Details

time,h      cp,mg/l      xd,mg         xm,mg          xu,mg     response

   .25        2.74        65.44          23.95          .73        +
   .50        3.40       128.92          57.08         1.75        +
   .75        1.25       120.23          73.02         2.24        -
  1.00        1.12       107.50          85.84         2.63        -
  1.25        1.00        96.12          97.30         2.98        -
  1.50         .89        85.94         107.55         3.29        -
  2.00         .72        68.70         124.90         3.83        -
  3.00         .46        43.90         149.86         4.59        -
  4.00         .29        28.05         165.81         5.08        -
  6.00         .12        11.46         182.52         5.59        -

AREA UNDER THE CURVE

The late time elimination constant is   .4478 1/h
The half life based on the last 3 points is     1.55 h
The extrapolation term is      .27 hour.mg/litre
The estimate of total area is       4.53 hour.mg/litre
```

The *C,t* plot of the results is shown in *Figure 5.1*. It is seen that the target plasma level of 4 mg/l is almost reached at 8 h; the active level is attained at 1 h.

The next runs are to evaluate a loading dose infusion schedule to use with this maintenance dose so as to reduce the time taken for the drug to reach an active plasma concentration.

In the simulation program the first infusion is given as a total dose over a specified period while the second infusion is expressed as a rate over a defined period. A loading dose of 100 mg is given as the first infusion, over 0.02 h; the second, maintenance infusion is 175 mg/h for 12 h.

This regimen is tested with the run set out below.

```
Run details
```

```
Lignocaine, 100mg IV infusion over 0.02h, second
infusion, 175 mg/h for 12h;

start, primary display, graph;

display and print C,t plot;

restart same drug
```

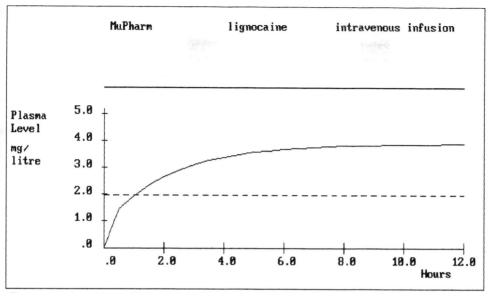

Press any key to continue

Figure 5.1 Lignocaine i.v. infusion 2100 mg/12 h (175 mg/h or 2.92 mg/min).

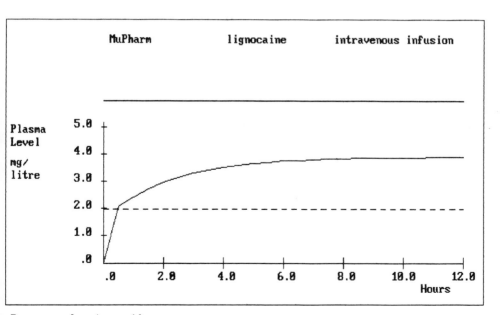

Press any key to continue

Figure 5.2 Lignocaine 100 mg/0.02 h + 175 mg/h i.v. infusion

The C,t plot is shown in *Figure 5.2*, the active level is reached at 0.4 h and the target level is almost attained in 7 h.

In an emergency, the period of 0.4 h before the active plasma level is reached would be too long; it is reduced by using a 200-mg loading dose. From *Figure 5.2*, the values of C are well below the toxic level and so a first infusion of 200 mg over 0.05 h is tested. Since it is only the early results which are of concern, the run time is reduced to 1 h, with results every 0.1 h.

```
Run details
```

```
Lignocaine, 200mg IV infusion over 0.05h, second
infusion, 175 mg/h for 1h;

run length 1h, 10 results at 0.1h intervals;

start, primary display, graph;

stop;

print results-log.
```

The numerical results from the results-log show that the active plasma level is reached before 0.1 h without a peak above the target level and therefore this regimen would be suitable for the emergency treatment of the standard subject.

2.4 Conclusions

The calculation of the infusion rate required to give an active, steady-state plasma concentration of a drug is straightforward, providing that the total clearance of the drug by the subject is known and that the drug disposition is first order, so that the clearance is independent of plasma concentration.

The calculated maintenance infusion may only produce active plasma levels of the drug quite slowly and it is often necessary to give a rapid loading dose before the maintenance infusion.

3. THE STEADY STATE WITH REPEATED ORAL DOSES

3.1 Calculations of the dose required to give a particular steady-state concentration

With the oral route, repeated doses are necessarily intermittent and a constant plasma level is not achieved. Between doses the plasma level fluctuations depend on a number of factors including the absorption rate, the plasma half-life and the biphasic kinetic behaviour of the drug.

The mean plasma concentration over the dosing interval increases, until it reaches a steady state in which the fluctuations over the dosing intervals are exactly repeated. A typical multi-dose C,t plot for a drug of short half-life is shown in *Figure 5.3*.

When the steady state is reached, the drug input exactly balances the elimination over the dosing interval. For many purposes it is convenient to use the mid-interval value of the plasma concentration C_{MI}, to assess the mean steady-state level.

The theory of the steady state for oral and i.m. doses is similar to that for i.v. infusion and has been outlined in Chapter 1, Section 11. If a dose D is given at intervals I_D, the amount of drug taken up in one dosing interval is $F \times D$, where F is the bioavailability of the drug. At the steady state this amount equals the amount eliminated, which is total clearance multipled by mean plasma concentration and by the dosing interval.

$$F \times D = Cl_T \times C_{SS} \times I_D$$

i.e.

$$D = Cl_T \times C_{SS} \times I_D/F$$

which is equation (1.14). This equation may be used to devise a dosing scheme which will result in achieving an appropriate target value for C_{SS} which is in the active range. The basis for deciding the value of I_D is discussed in Section 3.3.

The value of C_{SS} is decided in relation to the minimum active and toxic plasma levels of the drug; Cl_T and F are evaluated from single-dose studies with the drug and the subject and then D is calculated from the above equation.

3.1.1 *Alternative equation for calculating a repeated oral dose*

As shown in Chapter 1, Section 11, if the clearance in the above equation is expressed as $F \times D_1/\text{area}_T(D_1,\text{oral})$, where $\text{area}_T(D_1,\text{oral})$ is the total area under the C,t curve from a single oral dose D_1, the dose D to be given at intervals I_D to reach a target mean steady-state plasma concentration C_{SS} is (equation 1.15):

$$D = D_1 \times C_{SS} \times I_D/\text{area}_T(D_1,\text{oral})$$

This equation gives the same results as equation (1.14) without needing the value of F; it is useful in cases where the area following i.v. dose is not available or is difficult to determine.

3.2 **Effects on the steady state of enzyme induction and capacity-limited metabolism**

Steady-state calculations using equations (1.14) and (1.15) are based on the assumption of first-order disposition kinetics for the drug, resulting in a total clearance which is independent of plasma concentration. Since $Cl_T = F \times D/\text{area}_T$ by equation (1.12), constant clearance means that area under the C,t curve is proportional to dose. This property provides a good test for first-order kinetic behaviour.

With some drugs deviation from this behaviour occurs due to *enzyme induction* (Chapter 1, Section 6.6) which causes a slow increase in the rate of metabolism, resulting in an increase in the total clearance for a fixed repeated dose. In this case, after reaching an apparent steady state, mean plasma concentrations of drug begin to decline slowly over a long period.

Enzyme induction is a slow process; therefore in the first instance calculations of steady-state doses may be made with equations (1.14) and (1.15). With a schedule of repeated doses over a prolonged period, the induction effect may be counteracted by increasing the dose.

The anti-convulsant drug carbamazepine shows enzyme induction. In experiment 7, Section 6, the effect on steady-state plasma levels is shown.

Capacity-limited metabolism (Chapter 1, Section 6.1) may have a serious early effect on steady-state plasma concentrations. The capacity limitation means that clearance decreases as plasma concentration increases. At higher doses drug accumulation occurs, which may result in toxic plasma levels being reached.

The effects of this type of kinetic behaviour are discussed with experiments using phenytoin, in Chapter 7.

3.3 The dosing interval for repeated oral doses

The decision about the length of the dosing interval is made before the dose is calculated, on the pharmacokinetic basis of the drug half-life, and on clinical considerations such as the urgency of the condition being treated and the problem of patient compliance.

The pharmacokinetic basis is mainly concerned with the variation of plasma concentration over the dosing interval. If the half-life is short, this variation will be considerable and it is preferable to fix the interval at two half-lives or less, in order to ensure that plasma concentrations at the end of the half-life are still in the active range.

The urgency of the condition being treated is to some extent connected with the compliance problem. For example, consider ampicillin in the treatment of a severe case of acute bronchitis: the half-life is around 1.5 h, a 4- or 6-h dosing interval would therefore be appropriate and is unlikely to cause compliance problems while the patient is severely ill.

With a drug of short half-life, used for treatment over a long period, a short dosing interval would not be acceptable on the grounds of likely poor patient compliance. A longer interval than that indicated by the half-life is generally set. Alternatively, by using sustained release preparations, the dosing interval may be increased.

3.4 Time to reach the steady state

For planning runs to study repeated dosing schedules, it is advantageous to be able to calculate the length of a run required to reach the steady state. This problem is discussed mathematically in Appendix I, section 6.2; here the results are given for use in planning the repeated dose experiments.

For a maintenance dose, D, given at intervals I_D for N doses, the number of doses, N_{ss}, required to reach within say 1% of the steady state is a function of the half-life of the drug, $t_{1/2}$, and the dosing interval, I_D. The relationship is expressed by the inequality (I.30) renumbered (5.2):

$$N_{SS} > 6.65 \times t_{1/2}/I_D$$

(5.2)

The time from the start of dosing to within 1% of the steady state, t_{SS}, is given approximately by equation (I.31) renumbered (5.3) below:

$$t_{SS} = 6.65 \times t_{1/2} - I_D$$

(5.3)

3.5 Loading doses

Particularly with drugs of long half-life, the time taken for a maintenance dose alone to raise the plasma concentrations to a therapeutic level may be unacceptably long. In such cases, the first dose given is a loading dose which may be 2–4 times the maintenance dose. In order to avoid toxic effects, the loading dose is sometimes given in two or more divided portions, within the first dosing interval.

In order to determine a suitable loading dose using the simulation program, single-dose runs are made with trial doses with run lengths equal to the dosing interval. The ideal loading dose avoids toxic levels and gives an active plasma level at the end of the dosing interval which can be maintained by the following repeated doses.

The use of loading doses is important for repeated dosing with drugs which have capacity-limited metabolism. An example of simulation studies to establish a suitable loading dose for phenytoin is given in Chapter 7, Sections 4.4 and 4.5.

4. EXPERIMENT 6: ORAL MULTIDOSE REGIMEN FOR AMPICILLIN

In this experiment, ampicillin is used as an example for the calculation of a steady-state regimen of repeated oral dosing. This drug has first-order disposition kinetics and therefore the clearance is constant for a given subject.

4.1 Objective

The objective is to devise a repeated dosing schedule which will give plasma concentrations which reach an active level rapidly, and which maintain a steady-state plasma level of ampicillin in the active range and below the toxic level, with the standard subject.

4.2 Plan of experiment 6

For ampicillin the bioavailability and total clearance have been determined in Chapter 3, Section 2.3: $F = 0.481$ and $Cl_T = 11.7$ l/h. The half-life, 1.66 h, is short and a dosing interval of $I_D = 6$ h is chosen.

From Appendix II the minimum active plasma level is 2 mg/l and the toxic level is 30 mg/l. The target steady-state plasma level can therefore be set at 8 mg/l. The dose to be given every 6 h is then (from Chapter 1, Section 1.11, equation 1.14)

$$D = Cl_T \times C_{SS} \times I_D/F = 11.7 \times 8 \times 6/0.481 = 1168 \text{ mg}$$

In designing oral dose schedules it is advantageous to use standard doses and since the choice of mean target plasma level is not exact, the dose may be modified to some extent to comply with available preparations. This dose is therefore rounded to 1000 mg every 6 h.

With this dose the expected value of C_{SS} estimated from the ratio of rounded to calculated dose is:

$$C_{SS} = (1000/1168) \times 8 = 6.8 \text{ mg/l}$$

The length of a run to test this dosing regimen may be estimated; $t_{1/2}$ is 1.66 h and I_D is 6 h, the inequality (5.2) gives $N_{SS} > 1.84$, meaning that the steady state is reached at the second dose, consequently a run length of 24 h is suitable, with results every hour.

4.3 Runs and results

```
Run details



Ampicillin 1000mg every 6h for 4 doses, oral;

run length 24h, 24 results at 1h intervals;

standard subject;

start, primary display, graph;

display and print C,t plot.
```

The *C,t* plot is shown in *Figure 5.3*.

4.4 Conclusions

As can be seen, active plasma concentrations are rapidly reached and there is no need for a loading dose. Owing to the short half-life of ampicillin there is a wide variation of *C* within each dosing interval. However, the troughs remain above the minimum active level except for a short period at the end of each dosing interval and the peaks do not approach the toxic level: the regimen is therefore satisfactory. If necessary, the dosing interval could be reduced, to eliminate the sub-therapeutic plasma levels.

The mean value of *C* over the dosing interval is often approximated by the mid-interval *C* value C_{MI}. The values of C_{MI} may be obtained from the results-log and are shown below.

t (h)	3	9	15	21
C_{MI} (mg/l)	6.04	6.56	6.60	6.60

The steady state is reached at the third dose with C_{MI} close to the target of 6.8. No further run is required in this experiment, and so the program is stopped and the results-log is printed.

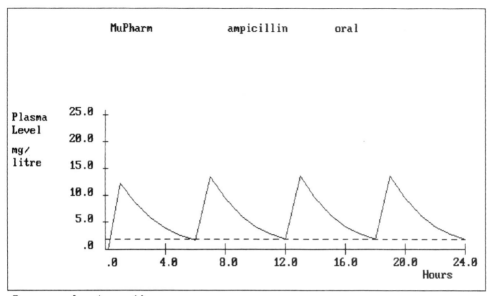

Press any key to continue
Figure 5.3 Ampicillin 1000 mg/6 h oral.

5. PEAK AND TROUGH PLOTS FOR MULTIPLE DOSING

With drugs of short half-life, there is a considerable change in plasma concentration over a dosing interval and the peak and trough concentrations are often more important than the mean steady-state level. An efficient plot for multiple dosing is a semilog graph showing just the peak and trough C values for each dosing interval. This plot indicates clearly any crossing of the toxic level line at the peaks and any crossing of the active level line at the troughs. The proportion (if any) of the dosing interval for which plasma concentrations are below the therapeutic level may be quantitatively estimated from this plot (Chapter 6, Section 6.3).

For the oral and i.m. routes, the peaks are generally taken as the C values 1 h after a dose is given, with troughs at the time at which the next dose is due. With sustained release preparations and with drugs which are only slowly absorbed, a later time should be taken for the peaks. For i.v. bolus doses, the peak is often taken as the C value at 0.25 h after dose. With repeated short i.v. infusions, the peak is generally at the end of each infusion period.

When a mean steady-state plasma level is satisfactory but the peaks are in the toxic range, the dose will have to be reduced; when the troughs are unsatisfactorily below the active level, the dose may be increased or the dosing interval be reduced.

113

6. EXPERIMENT 7: ORAL MULTIDOSE REGIMEN FOR CARBAMAZEPINE

6.1 Objective

Carbamazepine is an anti-convulsant drug which is often used for long-term treatment. The object of this study is to develop a suitable multidose scheme for long-term therapy. This drug induces the enzymes which cause its metabolism and the effect of this enzyme induction on the steady-state plasma levels is noted.

6.2 Plan

From Appendix II, the half-life of carbamazepine is 35 h, the active level is 4 mg/l and the toxic level is 10 mg/l.

In order to use equation (1.15) to calculate the repeated dose required for a suitable regimen for the standard subject, a single oral dose run for the estimation of $area_T$ is first made. An appropriate dose (Appendix II) is 200 mg. The run length is 120 h with 19 suitably spaced results.

In view of the long half-life, a dosing interval of 24 h is used. The target steady-state mean plasma concentration is chosen as 7 mg/l, midway between active and toxic levels. With these values and equation (1.15), the dose to be repeated every 24 h is evaluated.

$$D = I_D \times C_{SS} \times D_1 / area_T(D_1, oral)$$

(1.15)

The time to reach the steady state is calculated from equation (5.3):

$$t_{SS} = 6.65 \times t_{1/2} - I_D = 6.65 \times 35 - 24 = 209 \text{ h}$$

A long run of 240 h is therefore used with peak and trough results for each of the 10 dosing intervals. A semilog plot is chosen for the final display.

6.3 Runs and results

The run for area estimation is set up as outlined below.

```
Run details


Carbamazepine 200mg oral;

run length 120h, 19 results at 0.25, 0.5, 0.75, 1, 1.25,
1.5, 2, 3, 4, 6, 8, 12, 18, 24, 36, 48, 72, 96, 120h;

standard subject;

start, primary display, graph; area estimate;
```

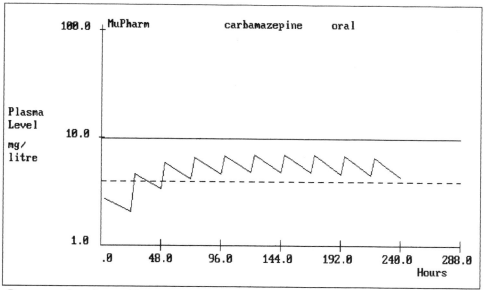

Press any key to continue

Figure 5.4 Carbamazepine 320 mg/24 h, peak and trough semilog plot.

From the area calculation, the value of k is 0.0197 h^{-1}, $t_{1/2}$ is 35.1 h, area$_T$ is 107.5 h mg/l; the area extrapolation term at 11.0 h mg/l indicates that the run has been of sufficient length.

The dose required to be given every 8 h to reach a target steady-state mean plasma concentration of 8 mg/l is estimated from equation (1.15).

$$D = D_1 \times C_{ss} \times I_D/\text{area}_T(D_1,\text{oral}) = 200 \times 7 \times 24/107.5 = 312.6 \text{ mg}$$

This dose is rounded to 320 mg/24 h and is tested in the next run which is made over 240 h. To reduce the number of results required, they are limited to peak and trough plasma concentrations for each interval. The peak is taken as 3 h after dose (the value of t_{max} in the single-dose study); the trough is the time of the next dose, just before it is given.

After restarting the program with the same drug there is no need to re-enter the subject details.

```
Run details



Carbamazepine, 320mg every 24h for 10 doses, oral;

run length 240h, 20 results at 3, 24, 27, 48, 51, 72, 75,
96, 99, 120, 123, 144h, 147, 168, 171, 192, 195, 216,
219, 240;
```

```
start, primary display, graph;

display and print semilog plot, auto minC and cycles;
```

The results are shown in *Figure 5.4*, from which it is seen that the active level is not reached until about 26 h after dose. Subsequently active levels are maintained throughout with a steady state being reached after the fifth dose at 96 h.

After the eighth dose at 168 h, the plasma levels begin to decline significantly, as a result of the enzyme induction. The numerical results are shown in *Table 5.2* which has an additional column showing the mean of the peak and trough values for each dosing interval.

The decrease in the mean C value is due to the fact that carbamazepine induces the enzymes which cause its metabolism. This enzyme induction means that the apparent elimination rate constant increases as time increases. Consequently, the clearance also increases with time.

The enzyme induction effect is the reason why the mean C values in *Table 5.2* are below the target of 7 mg/l.

Table 5.2 Carbamazepine, repeated doses.

```
****************** MUPHARM RESULTS-LOG *********************

Dose 320.00 mg of carbamazepine oral
repeated every 24.00 h for 10 doses

Numerical Details
```

time,h	cp,mg/1	Cmean	xd,mg	xm,mg	xu,mg	response
3.00	2.75		21.73	11.49	.73	−
24.00	2.08	2.42	110.46	98.98	6.47	−
27.00	4.70		134.61	121.15	7.88	+
48.00	3.42	4.06	213.63	270.83	17.48	−
51.00	5.94		234.27	300.52	19.32	+
72.00	4.23	5.09	286.07	492.89	31.30	+
75.00	6.67		302.81	527.75	33.39	+
96.00	4.67	5.67	330.51	748.82	46.72	+
99.00	7.04		344.22	787.17	48.95	++
120.00	4.86	5.95	354.38	1027.22	62.93	+
123.00	7.18		365.97	1067.94	65.22	++
144.00	4.91	6.05	364.37	1320.36	79.40	+
147.00	7.18		374.55	1362.67	81.70	++
168.00	4.86	6.02	365.38	1623.05	95.81	+
171.00	7.09		374.65	1666.46	98.08	++
192.00	4.75	5.92	360.80	1931.87	111.95	+
195.00	6.95		369.49	1976.03	114.17	+
216.00	4.61	5.78	352.86	2244.57	127.70	+
219.00	6.77		361.17	2289.27	129.87	+
240.00	4.45	5.61	342.99	2559.71	143.00	+

In order to reach active levels more rapidly, a loading dose could be given. However, loading doses are not generally used with carbamazepine; at the start of a course of treatment, the dose is built up gradually to the therapeutic level, so as to minimize adverse effects. For the same reason, the drug is often given every 12 h rather than at the 24-h intervals used in this study.

As this is the last run with carbamazepine, the program is stopped and the results-log is printed out.

6.4 Conclusions

A repeated dose regimen for carbamazepine based on calculations with equation (1.15) gives satisfactory plasma concentrations over a 240-h period. The enzyme induction effect causes mean plasma levels at the transient steady state to be lower than the target set. This effect also results in a reduction of the mean plasma concentration after 144 h. For long-term therapy, plasma levels of carbamazepine should be regularly monitored and the dose increased when necessary.

The enzyme induction causes a progressive decrease in the plasma half-life for carbamazepine: in the fifth dosing interval shown in *Figure 5.4*, $t_{1/2}$ is estimated as 36 h; in the tenth interval it has decreased to 31 h.

7. PROBLEMS

Use Appendix II to give the necessary information for setting up runs, including any single-dose runs necessary to determine area values. Use the standard subject in each case.

1. Evaluate a suitable continuous i.v. infusion to give constant therapeutic plasma concentrations of theophylline.
2. Design an i.v. bolus, repeated-dose regimen with benzylpenicillin for a patient (the standard subject) with life-threatening meningitis, using 2-hourly doses and keeping 0.25-h plasma concentrations as high as possible but below the toxic level.
3. Devise a repeated-dose regimen for phenobarbitone by the oral route.

CHAPTER 6

Multiple Dosing Regimens, Sustained-release Oral and Intramuscular Route. Studies with Oxprenolol and Benzylpenicillin

1. SUSTAINED-RELEASE DOSAGE FORMS

1.1 Introduction

Sustained release preparations are used for drugs which are given at frequent intervals and which are eliminated rapidly. An example is the beta-blocker oxprenolol, which may be used as a long-term treatment for hypertension.

An ideal preparation would, like an i.v. infusion, give a constant release rate for the drug, continuing for a long period and maintaining an active plasma level.

A number of methods have been proposed for developing sustained-release dosage forms, from which the drug is slowly released into the gastro-intestinal tract (GIT), e.g. the absorption of a drug into an insoluble gel such as an ion-exchange resin, or the use of a wax or polymer matrix.

1.2 Coating method for preparing sustained-release dosage forms

Coating methods have proved to be generally effective. In these methods, crystals or aggregates of solid drug are coated in an air suspension process, by an inert polymer of high molecular weight. The product is mixed with excipients and is compressed into tablets. The tablets are then coated overall with a semipermeable film which reduces the early release rate.

Detailed *in vitro* studies of coated tablets of oxprenolol indicate that the dose is released more rapidly at first, followed by a decreased rate of release. The rates of release are almost independent of pH and of surface tension. The polymer used is not digested and so the enzymes of the GIT do not affect the release rate.

1.3 Osmotically driven slow-release preparations

A development which extends the duration of release is the osmotically driven type of sustained-release preparation (Oros, Alza Corporation), in which the drug release is controlled by an osmotic pressure gradient. The solid drug is enclosed in a continuous, inert, semipermeable membrane in which there is a single, laser-drilled hole.

When the preparation enters the GIT, water permeates through the membrane and starts to dissolve the drug, which forms a saturated solution inside the membrane. The osmotic pressure difference between this solution and the gastro-intestinal fluid causes a further inflow of water; to make room for the water, drug solution is expelled through the hole.

So long as solid drug remains, the drug solution is saturated and the osmotic pressure difference is constant, giving constant rates of inflow of water and of outflow of solution. After about half of the drug has been delivered, the drug inside the membrane becomes completely dissolved and subsequent inflow of water lowers the solution concentration and the osmotic pressure difference. Consequently, a second, lower rate of release occurs.

2. PARAMETERS FOR SUSTAINED-RELEASE PREPARATIONS

In practice sustained release preparations only give a constant rate of release for a few hours; subsequent release continues at a decreased rate.

In the simulation model, oral sustained release is represented by two consecutive constant-rate (zero-order) processes. Two parameters, T_1 and T_2, define the durations of these processes; a third parameter, G, defines the proportion of the effective oral dose of drug which is released in the first process; a fourth parameter is the effective oral dose, D_{EO}, which is often less than the amount of drug contained in the preparation. The amount of drug included in D_{EO} is subject to the factors such as incomplete absorption and the first-pass effect, which cause the bioavailability of any oral dose of the drug to be less than one.

Sustained-release dosage forms generally show a lag time of around 1 h, during which no significant release occurs. *Figure 6.1* illustrates the representation for sustained release, used in the simulation. The area of each rectangle in *Figure 6.1* (equal to a constant rate of release multiplied by the time during which this rate operates), is equal to the amount of drug released during the corresponding period of the process.

The first release process starts at the end of the lag time and is set to end when the plasma concentration, as found experimentally, begins to decrease sharply; the end of the second process can sometimes be seen as a sharp drop in plasma concentration at a later time.

The effective oral dose is calculated from areas under the plasma-concentration–time curve; this area for the sustained-release preparation is compared with that for the same subject with the same amount of drug given by the oral route, in a conventional dosage form.

Sustained-release preparations usually show lag time effects and an estimate of lag time may be made from the first points in the data, as in Chapter 3, Section 2.3, Figure 3.1.

3. PARAMETER VALUES FOR A COATED-TABLET SUSTAINED-RELEASE PREPARATION

For the simulation model, it is useful to have a generally applicable set of parameters for the coated type of sustained-release preparation. They need to be used with caution, however, because results with individual subjects may differ markedly from those predicted with these general parameters. In *Table 6.1* a set of parameters is given.

Table 6.1 Parameters for a coated tablet sustained release preparation containing a total of *D* mg of drug.

Parameter	Symbol	Unit	Coated particle
Effective oral dose	D_{EO}	mg	$0.9 \times D$
Lag time	t_{lag}	h	0.7
1st release time	T_1	h	4
2nd release time	T_2	h	7
Fraction to 1st	G	–	0.7

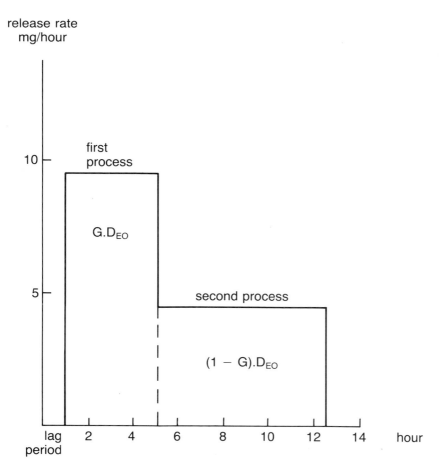

Figure 6.1 Rate of release, time plot, simulation model.

The drug used as an example in this chapter is oxprenolol and a summary of its properties is given in Appendix II.

4. EXPERIMENT 8: DESIGN OF MULTIPLE-DOSING REGIMENS WITH CONVENTIONAL AND SUSTAINED-RELEASE DOSAGE FORMS OF OXPRENOLOL

4.1 Objectives

The objectives are to devise dosage regimens for both conventional and sustained-release dosage forms of oxprenolol, so as to provide effective therapy for hypertension, with the standard subject.

4.2 Plan for area estimations

The half-life of oxprenolol is around 1.5 h and the dosing interval for a conventional oxprenolol tablet is 8 h; with an ideal sustained-release preparation this interval would be increased to 24 h.

First, estimations of the areas under the C,t curves are made from the results of runs with single doses of oxprenolol. From the areas the total clearance and bioavailability are calculated.

Two runs are made, one with a single i.v. infusion and the other with an oral dose. Information required for planning these runs is obtained from Appendix II. In view of the half-life, 12-h runs for area are suitable.

The two runs can be set up in succession so that the times for results need only be entered once. The doses used are 20 mg over 0.5 h for the i.v. infusion and 80 mg for the oral dose.

The plans for the repeated dose regimens are discussed after the area results have been obtained.

4.3 Area estimation runs and results

The two runs are set up in succession, as outlined below. At the end of the second run the program is stopped and the results-log is printed out.

```
Run details



Oxprenolol 20mg IV infusion over 0.5h;

run length 12h, 12 results at 0.25, 0.5, 0.75, 1, 1.25,
1.5, 2, 3, 4, 6, 8, 12h;

standard subject;

start, primary display, graph;
```

```
area estimation;

restart same drug;
```

At the end of this run, the oral dose run is set up. In this second run there is no need to reset the times or the subject as they are the same as in the previous run.

Table 6.2 Oxprenolol, area estimation.

```
******************* MUPHARM RESULTS-LOG **********************

Dose 20.00 mg of oxprenolol  intravenous infusion
1st infusion .50 h, 2nd infusion .00 mg/h for .00 h

Numerical Details

time       cp,microg/1    xd,mg     xm,mg     xu,mg      response

    .25      532.91         5.65      2.38       .05       +
    .50      644.17        11.73      5.82       .13       +
    .75      211.44        11.58      7.49       .17       +
   1.00      190.60        10.45      8.67       .20       +
   1.25      172.00         9.43      9.73       .22       +
   1.50      155.21         8.51     10.69       .25       +
   2.00      126.40         6.93     12.33       .28       +
   3.00       83.83         4.59     14.76       .34       +
   4.00       55.59         3.05     16.38       .38       -
   6.00       24.45         1.34     18.15       .42       -
   8.00       10.75          .59     18.94       .44       -
  12.00        2.08          .11     19.43       .45       -

AREA UNDER THE CURVE

The late time elimination constant is .4107 1/h
The half life based on the last 3 points is 1.69 h
The extrapolation term is 5.06 hour.microg/litre
The estimate of total area is 848.39 hour.microg/litre

Dose 80.00 mg of oxprenolol  oral

Numerical Details

time       cp,microg/1    xd,mg     xm,mg     xu,mg      response

    .25      418.21         3.83      6.34       .04       +
    .50      448.83         8.46     13.93       .10       +
    .75      455.63        11.76     20.71       .16       +
   1.00      452.45        13.99     26.75       .22       +
   1.25      442.08        15.39     32.13       .28       +
   1.50      426.57        16.15     36.94       .34       +
   2.00      386.27        16.33     45.07       .45       +
   3.00      294.78        13.99     56.81       .63       +
   4.00      212.79        10.69     64.41       .77       +
   6.00      102.19         5.41     72.62       .93       +
   8.00       46.67         2.52     76.17      1.01       -
  12.00        9.25          .51     78.40      1.06       -

AREA UNDER THE CURVE

The late time elimination constant is .4010 1/h
The half time based on the last 3 points is 1.73 h
The extrapolation term is 23.07 hour.microg.litre
The estimate of total area is 2003.91 hour.microg/litre
```

```
oxprenolol 80mg, oral;

start, primary display, graph;

area estimation;

stop;

print results-log.
```

The results of the runs and of the area estimations are shown in *Table 6.2*. From the 20-mg i.v. infusion run, the value of k is 0.411 h^{-1}, $t_{1/2}$ is 1.69 h; area$_T$ is 848 h µg/l or 0.848 h mg/l. From the 80-mg oral dose, k is 0.401 h^{-1}; $t_{1/2}$ is 1.73 h; area$_T$ is 2004 h µg/l or 2.00 h mg/l.

From the relative values of X_m (78.4 mg) and X_u (1.1 mg) at 12 h, for the oral dose, it is seen that oxprenolol is mainly eliminated by metabolism and that the fraction absorbed from the dose, F_a is almost equal to 1.0. The bioavailability of oxprenolol from the oral dose is (from equation 3.1)

$$F = \text{area}_T(80 \text{ mg,oral})/[4 \times \text{area}_T(20 \text{ mg,i.v.})] = 2.0/[4 \times 0.848] = 0.59.$$

Since oxprenolol is well absorbed from a conventional tablet, the low bioavailability is due to a substantial first-pass effect, as with nortriptyline (Chapter 3, Section 2.3).

The total clearance from the oral dose is (cf. Chapter 1, Section 10.3, equation 1.12)

$$Cl_T = F \times D/\text{area}_T(D,\text{oral}) = 0.59 \times 80/2.0 = 23.6 \text{ l/h}$$

The volume of distribution is best estimated from the i.v. results using equation (1.9) (Chapter 1, Section 9.5):

$$V = D/[k \times \text{area}_T(\text{i.v.})] = 20/[0.411 \times 0.848] = 57.4 \text{ l}$$

4.4 Plan for the conventional tablet regimen

The minimum active plasma concentration for oxprenolol is 0.06 mg/l and the minimum toxic level is 3 mg/l, giving a relatively high therapeutic ratio.

Because of the problem of patient compliance in the long-term therapy required, and the lasting duration of action of this group of drugs compared with their plasma half-lives, a comparatively long dosing interval of 8 h is used, $I_D = 8$ h. A target level of four times the minimum active level is chosen; $C_{SS} = 4 \times 0.06 = 0.24$ mg/l.

The estimate for the 8-hourly dose is then given by equation (1.14):

$$D = Cl_T \times C_{SS} \times I_D/F = 23.6 \times 0.24 \times 8/0.59 = 76.8 \text{ mg}$$

This value is rounded to 80 mg every 8 h.

Since the half-life is short, a loading dose is unlikely to be required and the steady state should be reached quite quickly. In order to test the scheme, the run is made for 48 h with peak and trough plasma concentration values.

4.5 Conventional tablet regimen. Runs and results

In the last run, the program was stopped to print the results-log, therefore this run has to be entered in full.

```
Run details
```

```
Oxprenolol 80mg every 8h, 6 doses, oral;
```

```
run length 48h, 12 results, 1, 8, 9, 16, 17, 24, 25, 32,
33, 40, 41, 48h;
```

```
standard subject;
```

```
start, primary display, graph;
```

```
display and print semilog plot, auto minC and cycles;
```

```
restart same drug.
```

The semilog plot is shown in *Figure 6.2*.

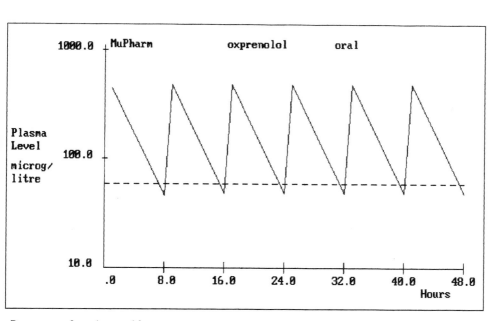

```
Press any key to continue
```

Figure 6.2 Oxprenolol 80 mg/8 h, oral.

As is seen, the values of C go below the active concentration (horizontal dotted line) right at the end of each dosing interval.

Like other beta-blockers, oxprenolol is firmly bound to the receptors which mediate its effect, consequently the effect persists longer than would be expected from the plasma levels. These short periods below the active level are unlikely to affect the continuity of the therapeutic effect. If considered necessary, the dose could be increased. However, this run does give a satisfactory dosing schedule.

4.6 Plan for the sustained-release regimen

As described in Chapter 6, Section 2, two constant-rate release processes are used as the kinetic model for sustained release in the simulation program. For a multi-dose regimen, the dose to be repeated is calculated from the target plasma level by setting the second, slower rate of release equal to the estimated elimination rate at C_{SS}.

Using the notation of Chapter 6, Section 3, the amount of the effective oral dose of the drug released in the second process is $(1 - G) \times D_{EO}$ mg. The amount of drug which reaches the plasma intact is this quantity multiplied by the bioavailability from the oral dose, F.

The time of release is T_2 h, and the rate of release is therefore $(1 - G) \times D_{EO}/T_2$ mg/h. The estimated rate of elimination at the target plasma level C_{SS} mg/l is $C_{SS} \times Cl_T$, where Cl_T is the total clearance, which is 23.6 l/h (Chapter 6, Section 4.3).

Introducing the bioavailability ($F = 0.59$) the rate at which intact drug reaches the plasma in the second release period is the bioavailability F times the effective dose D_{EO}, times the fraction going to the second release process $(1 - G)$ and divided by the duration of the second process T_2:

$$\text{rate}(X)_{uptk} = F \times D_{EO} \times (1 - G)/T_2 \text{ mg/h}$$

At the steady state, this rate is equal to the mean rate of elimination, which is the clearance Cl_T, multiplied by the target mean steady-state concentration, C_{SS}:

$$F \times D_{EO} \times (1 - G)/T_2 = Cl_T \times C_{SS}$$

on rearranging:

$$D_{EO} = Cl_T \times C_{SS} \times T_2/[(1 - G) \times F]$$

$$(6.1)$$

The target level is set at twice the minimum active level, because the sustained release reduces the change of plasma concentrations over the dosing interval, $C_{SS} = 0.12$ mg/l. Substituting values of G and T_2 for the general coated-particle preparation given in *Table 6.1* ($G = 0.7$, $T_2 = 7$ h):

$$D_{EO} = 23.6 \times 0.12 \times 7/(0.3 \times 0.59) = 112 \text{ mg}$$

From *Table 5.1*, the amount of oxprenolol required in the preparation, D, is $D_{EO}/0.9 = 112/0.9 = 124$ mg.

The calculated figure for oral doses may have to be adjusted to comply with available preparations. A standard sustained-release preparation for oxprenolol contains 160 mg and so for this study the value of D is taken as 160 mg.

The dose which is entered when the run is set up is

$$D_{EO} = 0.9 \times 160 = 144 \text{ mg}$$

The dosing interval may be assessed from the general release periods given in *Table 6.1*, $T_1 = 4$, $T_2 = 7$ h. Active plasma levels will thus be maintained for 11 h, and so taking in the lag time 0.7 h, a 12-h dosing interval is chosen.

In summary, the dose (D_{EO} for the simulation) is 144 mg repeated at 12-h intervals; the method of administration is oral sustained release; the first release period is 4 h and the second is 7 h; the fraction released in the first period is 0.7; the lag time is 0.7 h.

A run of 72 h, i.e. six dosing intervals, is suitable. The peak and trough plot is not used in this case and results are taken every 2 h, so that the sustained release effect may be seen.

4.7 Sustained-release regimen. Runs and results

The details for setting up the run are shown below.

```
Run details
```

```
oxprenolol 144mg every 12h for 6 doses, sustained release
oral, first release period 4h, second period 7h, fraction
to first 0.7;

run length 72h, 36 results at 2h intervals;

change, lag time to 0.7h;

start, primary display, graph;

display and print semilog plot, minC = 10, cycles = 2;
```

The semilog plot is shown in *Figure 6.3*.

The C values are above the active level, the troughs being well above this level. The sustained-release effect is shown by the shapes of the plot between doses.

4.8 Release pattern for the preparation

The release of oxprenolol from the sustained-release preparation may be estimated from the values of the four parameters D_{EO}, G, T_1 and T_2. D_{EO} is 144 mg and G is 0.7, therefore the amount released in the first process is $0.7 \times 144 = 101$ mg, the period of release is 4 h and therefore the rate of release is 25.2 mg/h.

The amount released in the second process is $0.3 \times 144 = 43$ mg over a period of 7 h, i.e. a rate of 6.2 mg/h.

The overall release pattern is, with time reckoned from the time of dosing:

0–0.7 h, lag time, no release
0.7–4.7 h, release rate 25.2 mg/h, amount 101 mg
4.7–11.7 h, release rate 6.2 mg/h, amount 43mg
Total amount released, 144 mg

These results are shown plotted as cumulative amount released against time, in *Figure 6.4.*

4.9 Conclusions

Oxprenolol has a bioavailability from an oral dose of around 60% due to a considerable first-pass effect. With the standard subject a regimen with repeated conventional tablets containing 80 mg of oxprenolol given every 8 h is adequate.

With the sustained-release preparation containing 160 mg of oxprenolol and given every 12 h, the trough plasma concentrations are well above the minimum active level. A reduced dose in the sustained-release preparation would give effective levels since this preparation reduces the fluctuations due to the short half-life of the drug, seen with the conventional tablet.

5. THE STEADY STATE WITH REPEATED INTRAMUSCULAR DOSES

The steady-state theory for a drug given by the i.m. route is similar to that for the oral route (Chapter 5, Section 3). The bioavailability used is that for the i.m. dose and the area under the curve for calculating clearance is estimated for this route.

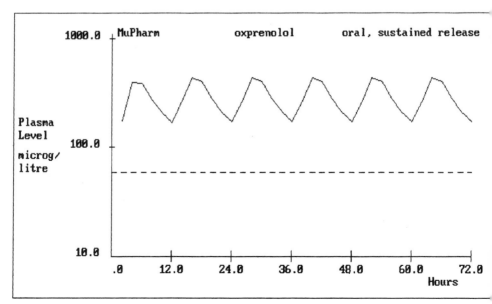

Press any key to continue

Figure 6.3 Oxprenolol 144 mg/12 h, oral sustained release.

cumulative amount
released, mg

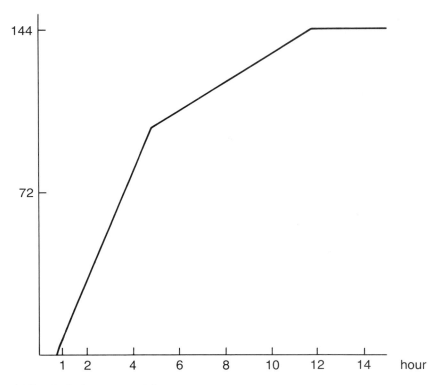

Figure 6.4 Sustained release, oxprenolol.

6. EXPERIMENT 9: REPEATED-DOSING REGIMEN FOR BENZYLPENICILLIN BY THE INTRAMUSCULAR ROUTE

Benzylpenicillin is taken as an example. This antibiotic, used for the treatment of bacterial infections such as pneumonia, diphtheria and forms of meningitis, cannot be administered by the oral route since its activity is greatly reduced by the acid conditions in the stomach.

6.1 Objective

The objective is to devise a regimen for treating the standard subject, suffering from a bacterial infection, with repeated i.m. doses of benzylpenicillin so as to maintain a plasma concentration of 2 mg/l of the drug.

6.2 Plan

From Appendix II, the half-life is around 1 h, the minimum active plasma concentration is 2 mg/l and the toxic level is 100 mg/l.

Equation (1.15) (renumbered 6.2 below for the i.m. route) for estimating a repeated dose based on only one area determination, holds for the i.m. as well as for the oral route.

$$D = D_1 \times C_{SS} \times I_D / \text{area}_T (D_1, \text{i.m.})$$

(6.2)

An i.m. run to determine area is first made with a 200-mg dose of benzylpenicillin. In view of the short half-life a run of 6 h is sufficient.

For the multidose run, a 6-h dosing interval is used; a target mean plasma level of 4 mg/l, twice the minimum active concentration, is chosen; the dose to be repeated is then estimated. The time to reach the steady state will be short and a run of 24 h with peak and trough plasma concentrations is made.

6.3 Runs and results

```
Run details



Benzylpenicillin, 200mg IM;

run length 6h, 10 results, 0.25, 0.5, 0.75, 1, 1.25, 1.5,
2, 3, 4, 6;

standard subject;

start, primary display, graph;

area estimation;

restart same drug.
```

The results are shown in *Table 6.3*. From the 6-h values of X_m (28.9) and X_u (130.2), the main elimination route is seen to be by urinary excretion of unchanged drug, metabolism accounting for about 18% of the total; the elimination rate constant is 0.88 h^{-1}, the half-life is 0.79 h and the area under the C,t curve is 9.9 h mg/l.

Substituting numerical values into equation (6.2), the dose to be repeated every 6 h to give the target value of the mean C_{SS} is:

$$D = 200 \times 4 \times 6/9.9 = 485 \text{ mg}$$

This figure is rounded to 500 mg every 6 h.

Table 6.3 Benzylpenicillin i.m., area estimation.

```
****************** MUPHARM RESULTS-LOG *********************

Dose 200.00 mg of benzylpenicillin intramuscular

Numerical Details

time,h      cp,mg/l      xd,mg      xm,mg      xu,mg      response

   .25        6.70       10.75       3.31      14.92         +
   .50        6.20       21.85       8.06      36.34         +
   .75        5.09       27.09      12.14      54.72         +
  1.00        4.11       28.21      15.45      69.66         +
  1.25        3.31       26.97      18.12      81.69         +
  1.50        2.66       24.54      20.27      91.38         +
  2.00        1.72       18.65      23.39     105.42         -
  3.00         .72        9.12      26.70     120.34         -
  4.00         .30        4.06      28.08     126.55         -
  6.00         .05         .73      28.88     130.19         -

AREA UNDER THE CURVE

The late time elimination constant is .8794 1/h
The half life based on the last 3 points is .79h
The extrapolation term is .06 hour.mh/litre
The estimate of total area is 9.91 hour.mg/litre
```

The run time is 24 h, with peak and trough results. Both *C,t* amd semilog plots are needed for the discussion of the results made below. The semilog plot shows up better if a minimum *C* of 0.1 and three log cycles are used rather than the automatic scaling.

```
Run details



Benzylpenicillin 500mg every 6h, 4 doses, IM;

length of run 24h, 8 results, 1, 6, 7, 12, 13, 18, 19,
24h; start, primary display, graph;

display and print C,t graph;

display and print semilog plot minC 0.1, 3 cycles;
```

The peak and trough C,t plot is shown in *Figure 6.5*. As expected the steady state is rapidly reached at the second dose. The plot looks reasonably satisfactory although the trough values at the end of each interval are below the active level. However, there is a fallacy in this conclusion, as is shown by repeating the run with results every hour.

Peak and trough *C,t* plots where the points are joined by straight lines, as in *Figure 6.5*, are usually misleading. From this figure, the duration of inactive plasma levels appears to be about 14% of the dosing interval.

Another run is made with the same doses but with a detailed set of results taken every hour.

131

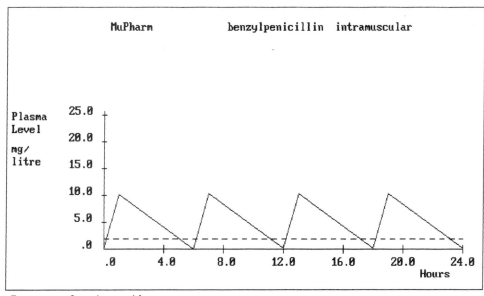

Press any key to continue

Figure 6.5 Benzylpenicillin 500 mg/6 h i.m.; peak and trough *C,t* plot.

```
Run details


length of run 24h, 24 results at 1h intervals

start, primary display, graph;

display and print C,t graph;

display and print semilog plot minC 0.1, 3 cycles;

reset same drug.
```

The *C,t* plot is shown in *Figure 6.6*. From this plot, the duration of inactive plasma levels is 52% of the interval — over three times the value from the peak and trough *C,t* plot. The reason for the discrepancy is that the lines joining the peak and trough values on the *C,t* plot are curved rather than straight as displayed in *Figure 6.5*.

The discrepancy can be resolved by considering *Figure 6.7*, in which the data of *Figure 6.6* are shown on a semilog plot. The lines joining the 1-h points on the plot are now straightened out, since the decline between peak and trough follows an approximately exponential relationship.

132

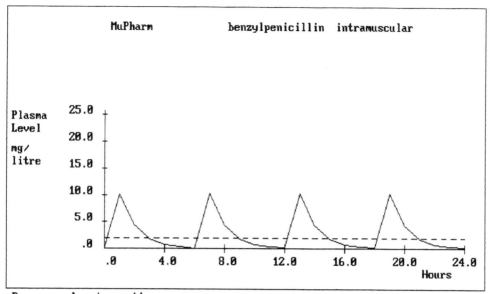

Press any key to continue

Figure 6.6 Benzylpenicillin 500 mg/6 h i.m.; results every hour; C,t plot.

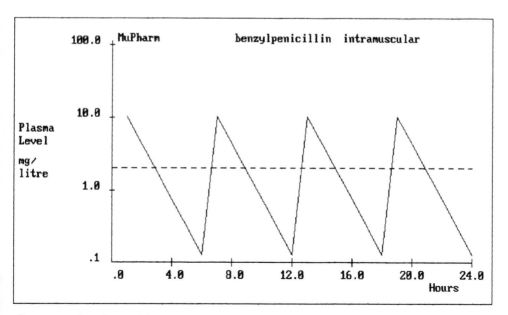

Press any key to continue

Figure 6.7 Benzylpenicillin 500 mg/6 h i.m.; results every hour; semilog plot.

The proportion of the later dosing intervals for which the plasma concentrations are inactive is estimated from this plot as 57%.

The semilog plot corresponding to the peak and trough data of *Figure 6.5* is shown in *Figure 6.8*, the straight lines are a much better representation of the intermediate concentrations than are the lines in *Figure 6.5*.

From *Figure 6.8*, the duration of the inactive plasma concentrations per interval is 57%, in agreement with the semilog plot value from the detailed, hourly results.

Whenever intermediate plasma concentration values are important, semilog plots should be used for peak and trough data.

6.4 Revised schedule for benzylpenicillin

The repeated-dose results in the run in Section 6.3 for benzylpenicillin are unsatisfactory because the plasma concentrations are below the active level for more than half of each dosing interval. By inspection of *Figure 6.8*, which is more reliable than *Figure 6.5*, it is seen that the plasma levels at 3 h after dose are at the active level.

For a further run a dose of 600 mg (a standard dose for this drug) every 3 h is given. This regimen is tested with a 24-h run.

The run details for the modified scheme are shown below. The prescription is altered and the times for results are changed to give peak and trough values for the 3-h dosing intervals. A semilog plot is chosen.

```
Run details


Benzylpenicillin 600mg every 3h for 8 doses, IM;

run length 24h, 16 results, 1, 3, 4, 6, 7, 9, 10, 12, 13,
15, 16, 18, 19, 21, 22, 24h;

start, primary display, graph;

display and print semilog plot, min C 0.1, cycles, 3;
```

The semilog peak and trough plot is shown in *Figure 6.9*. The C values are now above the minimum active level throughout, and the regimen is acceptable.

6.5 Conclusions

The short half-life of benzylpenicillin means that there is a large change in plasma concentration over a dosing interval of 6 h, and it would be difficult to maintain the relatively high active level of 2 mg/l used in this study over this period.

The misleading nature of *C,t* plots of peak and trough data has been shown; semilog plots should always be used for this type of data when assessment is required of the proportion of the dosing interval for which the plasma concentrations are below the active level.

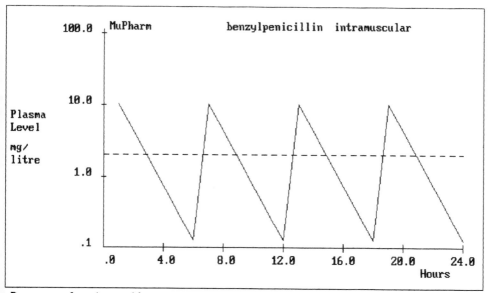

Press any key to continue

Figure 6.8 Benzylpenicillin 500 mg/6 h i.m.; peak and trough semilog plot.

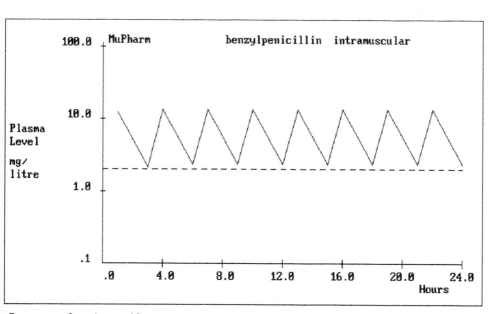

Press any key to continue

Figure 6.9 Benzylpenicillin 600 mg/3 h i.m.; peak and trough semilog plot.

135

In order to maintain active levels in this course of treatment, the dosing interval is reduced to 3 h and the dose is increased. It is the decrease of the interval which is the more important move for giving continuous active levels.

7. PROBLEMS

1. Make simulation model studies to determine areas under the curves for 25-mg doses of indomethacin (properties, Appendix II) given to the standard subject by i.v. infusion and by the oral route. Determine the total clearance, the volume of distribution and the bioavailability.
    Design and test a repeated oral dose scheme for the drug, given as a conventional preparation. Carry out a similar study with a sustained-release preparation of indomethacin having the characteristics summarized in Section 3.
2. Design an i.m. repeated-dose regimen with gentamicin similar to that for benzylpenicillin in experiment 9. Modify the repeated-dose scheme if necessary and re-run.

CHAPTER 7

Capacity-limited Metabolism and Repeated Dosing. Studies with Phenytoin

1. ENZYME KINETICS AND METABOLIC REACTIONS

Metabolic reactions which are catalysed by enzymes are governed by capacity-limited kinetics at higher substrate concentrations (Chapter 1, Section 6.1). When the starting concentration of the substance being metabolized (the substrate) is increased, the enzyme surface becomes saturated. Also, in conjugation reactions, available stocks of another reactant required may become depleted. In both cases, the reaction rate reaches a maximum value.

This type of kinetics is expressed by the Michaelis–Menten equation (Chapter 1, Section 6.1, equation 1.3):

$$\text{rate}(X) = -V_{max} \times C/(K_m + C)$$

where rate(X) is the rate of change in the amount X due to metabolism in mg/h, V_{max} is the maximum rate, also in mg/h; K_m is equal to the concentration at which the rate is $V_{max}/2$, in mg/l; C is concentration in mg/l; the sign is negative because the amount of drug X decreases as time increases.

As discussed in Chapter 1, Section 6.1, at low concentrations, the equation becomes that for a first-order process, with rate proportional to C. At high concentrations, the rate approaches $-V_{max}$, the process reaching complete saturation with a rate independent of C, thus becoming zero-order.

2. KINETICS OF DRUG DISPOSITION

The therapeutic plasma concentrations of most drugs are well below those associated with capacity limitation and their metabolism is effectively first-order. The elimination constant, k, is then independent of dose as is the total clearance, Cl_T; this may be considered to be ideal pharmacokinetic behaviour.

When the therapeutic plasma concentrations of a drug are in the range of capacity-limited effects, the drug exhibits positive deviation from the ideal. The apparent elimination constant decreases as the dose is increased, causing higher values of concentration than would be expected given first-order kinetics. Since in this case the total clearance varies with dose, clearance is not directly useful in estimating multi-dose schedules, equation (1.14) being only valid for first-order kinetics.

The saturable effect generally applies to elimination by metabolism; excretion of unchanged drug in the urine remains first order. The renal clearance is independent of concentration and therefore of dose, while the hepatic and total clearances decrease as the dose is increased.

With a potentially toxic drug such as phenytoin, the medical consequences of capacity-limited metabolism are serious. When repeated doses are given, the saturation effect may lead to a build-up of plasma concentrations so that toxic and possibly lethal levels of the drug are reached (Section 4.3).

Drugs such as carbamazepine (Chapter 5, Section 6.3), which induce their own metabolism, show negative deviation from the ideal; the apparent elimination constant increases with time, causing lower values of concentration than would be expected with first-order kinetics. The total clearance increases with time.

In this chapter phenytoin is taken as the example for developing multidose regimens with a drug showing saturable metabolism. The kinetic behaviour of this drug has been extensively studied since it is an important anticonvulsant with a low therapeutic ratio.

An experiment is first made with increasing single doses of phenytoin, to illustrate the method for detecting the plasma concentrations at which significant capacity-limited effects occur.

3. EXPERIMENT 10: THE DETECTION OF CAPACITY-LIMITED KINETICS. SINGLE-DOSE STUDIES WITH PHENYTOIN

3.1 Objective

Phenytoin (see Appendix II for details) is metabolized by saturable hydroxylation. The main objective of this experiment is to study the effects of the saturable metabolism on plasma concentrations in the therapeutic range.

3.2 Plan of the experiment

To perform this study, single-dose C,t runs are made with increasing doses of the drug. The C,t results from oral doses on either side of 400 mg are examined. The variations of the dose/area ratio and of the apparent plasma half-life with dose are assessed.

The high dose may be examined with the simulation model but would not be used in real studies, because of the risk of toxic effects at the resulting plasma concentrations.

The apparent half-life of phenytoin at low doses (100 mg) is around 11 h (Appendix II), increasing as the dose increases. For determining the area under the C,t curve, run times of 72 h are chosen, with plasma concentration results at 0.25, 0.5, 0.75, 1, 1.25, 1.5, 2, 3, 4, 6, 8, 12, 18, 24, 36, 48, 60 and 72 h — a total of 18 results.

The oral doses used in this experiment are 100, 400 and 1600 mg. In addition, a run with an i.v. infusion is made at the lowest dose of 100 mg, to give estimates of bioavailability and apparent volume of distribution.

The apparent half-life, which varies with concentration in the range of saturation of metabolism, is taken from the area estimations.

The runs are set to follow one another so that the timings and choice of subject do not have to be re-entered.

3.3 **Runs and results**

The dialogue for the four runs is set out below. For the three oral dose runs, semilog plots are printed out with the same minimum concentration (0.01), and the same number of cycles (4), so that they can be superimposed to give the composite diagram shown in *Figure 7.1*. For the i.v. infusion run, only the value of area is required.

```
Run details


Phenytoin 100mg oral;

run length 72h, 18 results, 0.25, 0.5, 0.75, 1, 1.25,
1.5, 2, 3, 4, 6, 8, 12, 18, 24, 36, 48, 60, 72h

standard subject;

start, primary display, graph;

area estimation;

display and print semilog plot, minC 0.01, 4 cycles;

restart same drug.

Phenytoin 400mg oral;

start, primary display, graph;

area estimation;

display and print semilog plot, minC 0.01, 4 cycles;

restart same drug.

Phenytoin, 1600mg oral;

start, primary display, graph;

area estimation;

display and print semilog plot, minC 0.01, 4 cycles;

restart same drug.
```

```
Phenytoin, 100mg IV infusion over 0.5h;

start, primary display, graph;

area estimation;

stop;

print results-log.
```

Figure 7.1 shows the three semilog plots of the *C,t* results for the 100-, 400- and 1600-mg oral doses of phenytoin. The plots show the change of shape caused by the limited-capacity kinetics. A drug with first-order elimination would give parallel linear plots at later times.

The 400-mg curve shows a shallower slope after 12 h than the 100-mg curve, indicating that the apparent elimination rate 'constant' is varying with dose. For the 1600-mg curve, the late time slope is shallower still.

From these plots it is seen that phenytoin is absorbed quite slowly from the oral doses, giving a maximum concentration at about 4 h after dose.

3.3.1 *Areas and apparent plasma half-lives*

In *Table 7.1* values of the apparent half-lives, the total areas under the *C,t* curves and the dose/area$_T$ ratios which are proportional to total clearances, are given for the three doses.

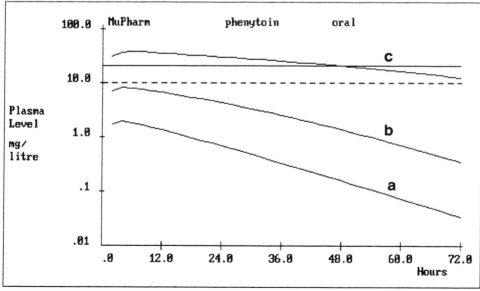

Press any key to continue

Figure 7.1 Phenytoin: (a) 100 mg oral (b) 400 mg oral; (c) 1600 mg oral.

140

Table 7.1 Kinetic parameters for oral phenytoin

Dose (mg)	Apparent $t_{1/2}$ (h)	area$_T$ (h mg/l)	dose/area$_T$ l/h
100	10.9	42.9	2.33
400	11.9	246	1.62
1600	33.1	2332	0.69

The apparent half life increases with increasing dose and the dose/area$_T$ ratio falls.

The 100mg i.v. infusion over one hour gives an area$_T$ value of 42.9 mg.h/l. The apparent bioavailability F, from an oral dose of 100mg, is therefore $42.9/44.9 = 0.955$, indicating almost complete absorption of phenytoin given by oral route.

3.3.2 *Volume of distribution*

The equation for calculating volume of distribution (Chapter 1, Section 9.5, equation 1.9) is only valid for drugs with first-order kinetics. It may be applied to the results from the 100-mg i.v. dose of phenytoin which are in a region far enough away from the saturation effect to give approximately first-order behaviour. The apparent elimination constant, from the i.v. area estimation, is 0.0634 h^{-1}; the apparent volume of distribution, using the i.v. infusion area, is

$$V = D/(k \times \text{area}_T) = 100/(0.0634 \times 44.9) = 35.1 \text{ l}$$

3.3.3 *Renal clearance*

Renal clearances may be assessed from equation (1.11):

$$Cl_r = (\text{rate of urinary excretion})/(\text{mean plasma concentration})$$

Taking the interval from 24 to 36 h in the 100-, 400- and 1600-mg dose results, the values shown in *Table 7.2* are obtained; D is dose in mg; ΔX_u is amount in mg excreted unchanged in the urine from 24 to 36 h; C_{mean} is the mean of the 24- and 36-h plasma concentrations in mg/l; rate $(X)_u$ is the mean rate of excretion, $\Delta X_u/12$ mg/h; Cl_r is rate $(X)_u/C_{mean}$; $X_{u,T}$ is the final value of X_u at 72 h and P_u is $100 \times X_{u,T}/D$, the percentage of the total dose which is excreted unchanged in the urine.

The renal clearance is substantially independent of dose and all the variation of total clearance is due to the hepatic clearance.

Although the renal clearance does not vary significantly, the percentage of the dose excreted unchanged in the urine increases as the dose increases. This is because the rate of urinary excretion in mg/h is equal to plasma concentration multiplied by renal clearance. Owing to the saturation of metabolism at higher concentrations, the plasma concentrations are far above the values expected from first-order kinetics.

Table 7.2 Renal clearances for phenytoin, 24 to 36 h

D (mg)	ΔX_u (mg)	$\text{rate}(X)_u$ (mg/h)	C_{mean} (mg/l)	Cl_r (l/h)	$X_{u,T}$ (mg)	P_u (%)
100	0.38	0.0317	0.51	0.062	2.65	2.7
400	2.63	0.219	3.52	0.062	15.1	3.8
1600	20.5	1.71	27.0	0.063	110.7	6.9

3.4 Approximate estimation of V_{max} and K_m

Approximate estimates of the Michaelis–Menten parameters may be made as follows. From the results-log, the 24- and 36-h values of C following the 100-mg dose are 0.69 and 0.33 mg/l respectively. The difference between these two values, 0.36, multiplied by the volume of distribution, 35.1 l, gives 12.6 mg as an approximate estimate of the amount of phenytoin eliminated over the 12-h period, corresponding to an elimination rate, rate $(X)_{e,1}$ of 12.6/12 = 1.05 mg/h. If the urinary excretion is ignored

$$\text{rate } (X)_{e,1} = V_{max} \times C_1/(K_m + C_1)$$

(7.1)

where C_1 is the mean value of C over the interval, $C_1 = 0.51$ mg/l; the sign is positive because the amount eliminated increases as time increases.

The same calculations are made with the 24- to 36-h results following the 1600-mg dose; at 24 h, $C = 29.35$ and at 36 h, $C = 24.62$ mg/l. The mean rate is

$$\text{rate } (X)_{e,2} = (29.35 - 24.62) \times 35.1/12 = 13.8 \text{ mg/h}$$

the mean concentration is 27.0 mg/l.

Substituting the two pairs of values of rate and C into the Michaelis–Menten equation:

$$1.05 = V_{max} \times 0.51/(K_m + 0.51)$$

$$13.8 = V_{max} \times 27.0/(K_m + 27.0)$$

The second equation is divided by the first to give an equation for K_m, and on carrying out the arithmetic

$$K_m = 8.23 \text{ mg/l}$$

Substituting this value into the second equation gives

$$V_{max} = 18.0 \text{ mg/h}$$

These values are approximate because the urinary excretion of unchanged drug has been neglected.

4. EXPERIMENT 11: THE DEVELOPMENT OF A LONG-TERM MULTI-DOSE REGIMEN FOR PHENYTOIN

4.1 Objective

The objective of this experiment is to devise an oral dosing schedule with the standard subject which will give active levels of phenytoin over a period of several weeks, with plasma concentrations below the toxic level.

4.2 Plan for regimen assuming first-order kinetics

In order to illustrate the perils of failing to recognize saturable effects with a potentially toxic drug, a multi-dose regimen for phenytoin is first evaluated assuming ideal first-order kinetics.

The preliminary work for the evaluation of an oral multi-dose scheme by the method of Chapter 5, Section 3.1, which assumes first-order kinetics, has been done in Section 3.3. The apparent plasma half-life for the 100-mg dose is 10.9 h and so a dosing interval, I_D, of 24 h is chosen.

The minimum active plasma concentration for phenytoin is 10 mg/l and the toxic level is 20, giving the small value of 2.0 for the therapeutic ratio. The target plasma level is taken as midway between these concentrations: 15 mg/l.

The required dose is now calculated from equation (1.15), assuming first-order kinetics. The values of D_1 and $area_T$ used are those for the oral dose of 400 mg.

$$D_T = D_1 \times C_{SS} \times I_D/area_T(D_1,PO) = 400 \times 15 \times 24/246 = 585 \text{ mg}$$

This dose is rounded to 600 mg every 24 h.

A run of 144 h with peak (4 h after dose), mid-interval (12 h after dose) and trough (24 h after dose) results is made, with presentation of results as a semilog plot.

4.3 Runs and results; first-order kinetics assumption

```
Run details



Phenytoin 600mg every 24h for 6 doses, oral;

run length 144h, 18 results, 4, 12, 24, 28, 36, 48, 52,
60, 72, 76, 84, 96, 100, 108, 120, 124 132, 144h;

standard subject;

start, primary display, graph;

display and print semilog plot, auto minC and cycles;

restart same drug.
```

The semilog plot is shown in *Figure 7.2*. The saturation effect is apparent from *Figure 7.2* which shows no sign of a steady state being reached. At the third dose, C goes above the toxic level, indicated by the full horizontal line on the graph. The mid-interval C values in mg/l are:

t (h)	12	36	60	84	108	132
C_{MI}	11.1	18.4	24.5	29.9	34.8	39.3

The apparent half-lives are proportional to the slopes of the plot within each dosing interval, and it can be seen that as the concentration rises and the saturation effect increases, these slopes become progressively shallower with each dose.

At very high concentrations, the first-order urinary excretion of unchanged drug will eventually balance the drug intake and a steady state will develop. The fate of the subject will depend on whether or not this balance occurs before the lethal plasma level of 70 mg/l is reached.

Figure 7.3 shows a semilog plot of the results from a continuation of the run for a further 6 days — the values of peak plasma concentrations are continuing to increase.

4.4 Plan for evaluating the doses

The problem of multiple dosing with a drug with saturable kinetic behaviour may be solved by starting with a loading dose which will take C up to the active level. A lower maintenance dose is then given at intervals, to keep C above the minimum active level and below the toxic level.

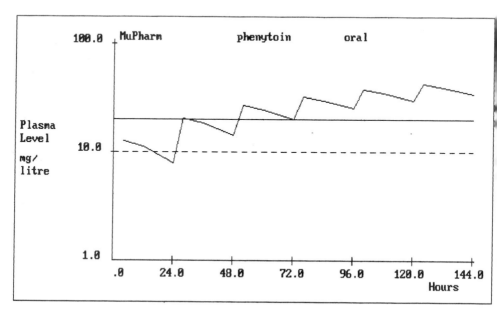

Press any key to continue

Figure 7.2 Phenytoin 600 mg/24 h; semilog plot.

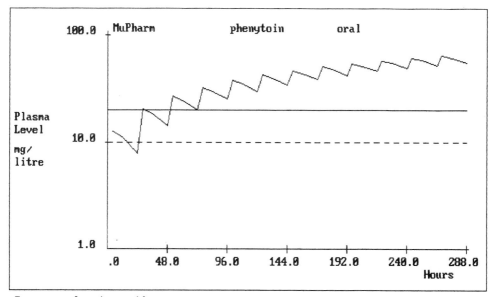

Press any key to continue

Figure 7.3 Phenytoin 600 mg/24 h, continued run; semilog plot.

A schedule of phenytoin maintenance doses suitable for the standard subject in the simulation model may be developed either by trial and error in the simulation model or from consideration of the approximate V_{max} and K_m values for this subject. The second method is outlined in Section 4.6.

A suitable loading dose is evaluated by making a series of 24-h runs with various single doses. A dose which gives a 24-h C value close to the minimum active level is chosen from these runs.

4.5 Runs and results; loading dose

The results of the first 24 h of the previous run may be taken as the first study to evaluate a suitable loading dose. The peak concentration at 4 h is 12.7, the mid-interval value at 12 h is 11.1 and the trough value at 24 h is 7.9 mg/l. The trough value is too far below the minimum active level of 10 mg/l and so two further single-dose 24-h runs are set up with single doses of 700 and 800 mg of phenytoin. The primary option chosen is the table of numerical results, the results being taken at 4, 12 and 24 h after each dose.

```
Run details


Phenytoin 700mg oral;

run length 24h, 3 results at 4, 12 and 24h;
```

```
start, primary display, table;

restart same drug.


Phenytoin 800mg oral;

start, primary display, table;

stop;

print results-log.
```

The 4-h peak, 12-h mid-interval and 24-h plasma concentration values are shown in *Table 7.3*. The values for the first 24 h of the 600-mg dose run are included.

The results in *Table 7.3* show that the 700-mg dose gives a trough value of C near the minimum active level of 10 mg/l. The peak value is satisfactory and therefore this dose is chosen as the loading dose for the next run.

4.6 Plan for the evaluation of a maintenance dose

The 600-mg/24-h dose of *Figure 7.3* is clearly much too large and a suitable maintenance dose to be given every 24 h may be estimated from the approximate values of V_{max} and K_m for the standard subject, calculated in Section 3.4.

According to equation (7.1), the mean rate of elimination of phenytoin at a mean steady-state plasma concentration of C_{SS} is

$$\text{rate}(X)_e = V_{max} \times C_{SS}/(K_m + C_{SS})$$

Assuming the steady state with doses D given at intervals I_D, the amount of drug eliminated over the dosing interval may be estimated as the mean rate multiplied by the interval. Then assuming that the dose is completely absorbed ($F = 1$):

$$\text{dose} = \text{amount eliminated in a dosing interval}$$

Table 7.3 Results from single-dose phenytoin runs

Dose (mg)		C (mg/l)	
	4 h (peak)	12 h (MI)	24 h (trough)
600	12.7	11.1	7.9
700	15.0	13.4	9.8
800	17.3	15.6	11.9

$$D = I_D \times \text{rate}(X)_e$$

therefore

$$D = I_D \times V_{max} \times C_{SS}/(K_m + C_{SS})$$

When the numerical values I_D = 24 h, V_{max} = 18.0 mg/h, K_m = 8.23 mg/l, C_{SS} = 15 mg/l (the units are correct for giving the required maintenance dose in mg) are substituted, we get

$$D = 24 \times 18.0 \times 15/(8.23 + 15) = 279 \text{ mg}$$

This value is rounded to 275 mg every 24 h.

In order to test the maintenance dose a run is made of length 144 h, with doses of 275 mg every 24 h and a loading dose of 700 mg, given in two portions at 12-h intervals. Peak, mid-interval and trough concentration values are recorded. The primary display is the table of results so that a dose alteration, if required, may be directly assessed at the end of the run from the screen.

4.7 Regimens with loading and maintenance doses. Runs and results

The first run is set up with a loading dose of 700 mg and a maintenance dose of 275 mg every 24 h.

Run details

```
Phenytoin 275mg every 24h, 6 doses oral, loading dose
700mg in 2 divided portions at 12h intervals;

run length 144h, 18 results at 4, 12, 24, 28, 36, 48, 52,
60, 72, 76, 84, 96, 100, 108h, 120, 124, 132, 144;

standard subject;

start, primary display, table;

restart same drug.
```

The mid-interval results, with C_{MI} in mg/l, are:

t (h)	12	36	60	84	108	132
C_{MI}	5.85	13.70	13.05	12.53	12.12	11.80

In the last interval the change in C_{MI} is – 0.32 mg/l.

The next run is made with an increased maintenance dose of 325 mg, and the same loading dose.

```
Run details
```

```
Phenytoin 325mg every 24h, 6 doses oral, loading dose
700mg in 2 divided portions at 12h intervals;
```

```
Start, primary display, table;
```

The results are:

t (h)	12	36	60	84	108	132
C_{MI}	5.85	14.83	15.09	15.31	15.49	15.63

C_{MI} increases by 0.14 over the last interval.

With the 325-mg/24-h dose, C_{MI} increases by 0.14 over the last interval and with the 275-mg/24-h dose, it decreases by 0.32; an intermediate value for the maintenance dose which would give a zero change over the last interval, may be estimated by proportion.

$$D = 275 + (325 - 275) \times 0.32/(0.32 + 0.14) = 310 \text{ mg}$$

However, for practical purposes a round figure value may have to be chosen and the safer alternative, so as to avoid possible toxicity, is 300 mg every 24 h. This value is used in the run set up below.

4.8 Plan for a long-term test for the phenytoin regimen

The prescription is 300 mg phenytoin every 24 h with a loading dose of 700 mg in two portions. In the first place a run of 144 h is made so that if the maintenance dose needs to be altered again, it may be done before the long run. If no alteration is required, the run is continued up to 576 h (24 days). The table of results is chosen as the primary display so that the mid-interval concentration value may be checked.

For the 144-h run, 18 results are taken, at 4, 12 and 24 h after each dose; the standard subject is used. These are the same timings and the same subject as in the previous run and so these details do not have to be re-entered. At the end of the run a semilog plot is displayed and printed.

4.9 Runs and results; long-term test

The run is set up as follows.

```
Run details
```

```
Phenytoin 300mg every 24h for 6 doses oral, 700mg loading
dose in 2 portions at 12h intervals;
```

```
start, primary display, table;
```

```
display and print semilog plot, auto minC and cycles;
```

```
restart same drug;
```

The semilog plot results are shown in *Figure 7.4*.

The loading and maintenance dose appear to be satisfactory and the run is continued three times with doses to give a total run time of 576 h (24 days).

It is convenient, with the simulation, to set up long runs in shorter portions (Chapter 4, Section 3.6). If a number of individual times for results are required, they only have to be entered for the first shorter run and they are then automatically copied in the continued run(s).

```
Run details
```

```
Continue, with doses;
```

```
Continue, with doses;
```

```
Continue, with doses;
```

```
display and print semilog plot, auto minC and cycles;
```

```
stop;
```

```
print results-log.
```

The semilog plot is shown in *Figure 7.5*; the earlier results are automatically added in, on continuation, giving a complete final plot of all the results.

4.10 Conclusions

Phenytoin shows marked saturable metabolism at plasma concentrations in the therapeutic range, the ratio of area under the C,t curve to oral dose decreases markedly at higher doses.

As a result of this effect, a dosing regimen based on a maintenance dose calculated on the assumption of first-order kinetics rapidly leads to toxic plasma levels of the drug.

A satisfactory regimen is obtained by using a loading dose to reach the therapeutic plasma level in the first interval, a maintenance dose is then estimated using the Michaelis–Menten equation or may be evaluated by trial and error.

The final scheme for the standard subject, 700 mg plus 300 mg every 24 h, gives plasma concentrations which are generally acceptable. It is seen from *Figure 7.4* that with the divided loading dose, an active plasma concentration is reached at the end of the first dose interval and apart from a brief dip below the active level at the end of the later intervals, therapeutic levels are maintained over the 24 days of the run with peaks well below the toxic level.

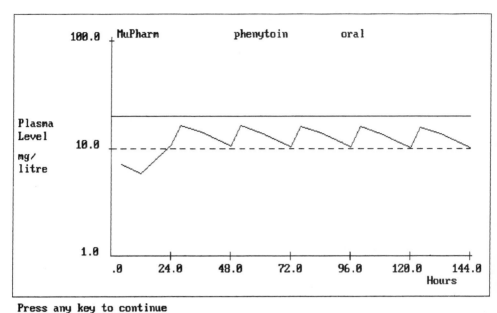

Press any key to continue

Figure 7.4 Phenytoin 300 mg/24 h oral, 700-mg loading dose in two portions at 12-h intervals.

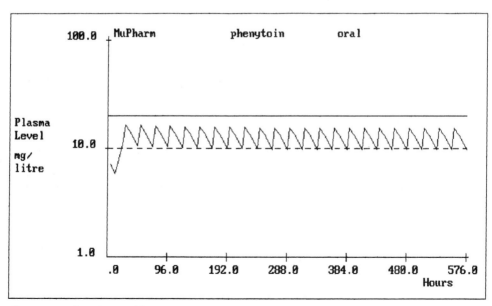

Press any key to continue

Figure 7.5 Run for *Figure 7.4* continued for 24 days.

150

Some mid-interval plasma concentrations in mg/l are:

t (h)	60	132	204	276	348	420	492	564
C_{MI}	14.1	13.7	13.5	13.4	13.3	13.3	13.3	13.3

With the saturation effect, it takes a long time for a steady state to become finally established.

The final dose interval values are, peak at 556 h, 15.42; mid-interval at 564 h, 13.25; trough at 576 h, 9.75 mg/l.

If the maintenance dose were to be increased to the value 310 mg, which was estimated by proportion, sub-therapeutic troughs would be avoided.

5. ASPIRIN

With the high doses which have been used in the treatment of rheumatic disease, aspirin shows limited-capacity metabolism. The metabolism of aspirin is complicated and has been represented in a simplified form in the simulation model.

Aspirin, acetyl-salicylic acid, is rapidly hydrolysed *in vivo* to salicylic acid, which is then further metabolized; the longer-term effects of dosage with aspirin are due to salicylate. Both acids are almost completely ionized at plasma pH values, and so the metabolites are given the names of their anions.

The further metabolism of salicylate has been studied by Levy, Tsuchiya and Amstel [*Clin. Pharmacol. Ther.*, (1972) **13**, 258] who found that with 2-g doses, 50% was excreted as salicylurate and 20% as a phenolic glucuronide. These two metabolites are both formed by capacity-limited processes.

In the simulation model, the kinetic scheme for aspirin is simplified by taking salicylurate and the phenolic glucuronide as the single metabolite; the drug is then total salicylate, i.e. acetyl-salicylate plus salicylate, and the plasma concentrations are the sum of the concentrations of these two substances which together give the therapeutic effect. Two minor metabolites formed by first-order processes are taken into the amounts of unchanged salicylate excreted in the urine.

6. PROBLEMS

1. Apply the dose/area test for saturable kinetics described in Section 3.3, to examine the overall kinetics of aspirin in the range of oral doses used for the treatment of acute rheumatic fever (the minimum active level in Appendix II). Take the central dose as 2000 mg with low and high doses of 500 and 5000 mg. Assess the apparent plasma half-lives and dose/area ratios for the different doses. Use the data in Appendix II to decide the run length.
    Determine the bioavailability and volume of distribution for the 500 mg dose by making an i.v. infusion run.

2. Use the methods described in this chapter to evolve a multi-dose scheme for aspirin in the treatment of rheumatic disease, using the standard subject. The minimum active and toxic levels are given in Appendix II. As in Section 4.2, assume first-order kinetics in the first place. Test the scheme and modify it until a satisfactory regimen is obtained.

CHAPTER 8

Pharmacokinetics in Disease States.
Studies with Paracetamol and Gentamicin

1. INTRODUCTION

In this chapter the effects of hepatic and renal dysfunctions on the pharmacokinetics of paracetamol and gentamicin are examined. The standard 70-kg male subject is used in the experiments described; in the next chapter the use of different subjects is explored.

Changes of functions are made in the dialogue of the simulation program by altering subject and drug factors. Full lists of the two sets of factors are given in Appendices III and IV.

The alterations considered in this chapter are to the subject parameters governing hepatic and renal functions.

Severe hepatic dysfunction may cause a reduction in the rate of metabolism of a drug; if metabolism is the main route of elimination the plasma half-life increases and there is drug accumulation. This effect can produce toxic plasma concentrations with drugs of low therapeutic ratio such as phenytoin (Chapter 7).

2. PARACETAMOL

Paracetamol, a drug which is mainly metabolized before excretion, is taken as the example in this experiment. The principal metabolites are the glucuronide and sulphate conjugates which account for 85% of a therapeutic dose; there is also a glutathione conjugate, accounting for 10%. After very high doses, such as those taken in suicide attempts, the conjugation pathways become saturated and an intermediate metabolite appears which is toxic to the liver and causes irreversible liver damage.

In cases of self-poisoning with paracetamol, the extent of liver damage may be assessed by determining the plasma half-life of the drug.

The minimum toxic plasma concentration for paracetamol is high at 120 mg/l and the active level is 5 mg/l. It is therefore comparatively safe in ordinary use.

3. EXPERIMENT 12: TO STUDY THE EFFECTS OF HEPATIC DYSFUNCTION ON THE PHARMACOKINETICS OF PARACETAMOL

3.1 Objectives

The objectives of the experiment are to study the effects of hepatic dysfunction on the plasma concentrations of paracetamol following single oral doses, and to devise repeated-dose regimens for the standard subject and for the same subject with a severe liver dysfunction.

3.2 Plan for single doses

To illustrate the effect on paracetamol plasma concentrations of increasing degrees of hepatic dysfunction, a series of runs are made with a 1000-mg oral dose given to the standard subject, with hepatic function values of 1.0, 0.7 and 0.4 (0, 30 and 60% reductions in function). Concentration values are taken every hour for 8 h.

In the simulation model, two subject factors govern hepatic function. The first, subject factor 5, is 1.0 for the standard 183-cm, 70-kg, 25-year-old male subject and is adjusted automatically in the program for other subjects; it cannot be altered interactively. The second, subject factor 6, has a value of 1.0 for normal hepatic function in all subjects and may be adjusted interactively to give changes in this function. For example, to produce a 60% reduction in function in any subject, this second factor would be altered to 0.4.

At the end of each run a semilog plot is chosen, each with the same minimum *C* and number of cycles, so that they can be compared as shown in *Figure 8.1*. A minimum *C* of 0.1 and four cycles are suitable for these runs.

3.3 Runs and results; single doses

The three runs are set up as described below.

```
Run details
```

```
Paracetamol 1000mg oral;

run length 8h, 8 results at 1h intervals;

standard subject;

start, primary display, table;

display and print semilog plot, minC 0.1, 4 cycles;

re-start same drug.
```

For the next run, the hepatic function, subject factor 6, sf(6), is changed to 0.7. The prescription and run details are not altered and at the end of the second run the semilog plot is again chosen. A restart with the same drug is selected and sf(6) is changed to 0.4 for the third run.

Run details

```
Change, sf(6) from 1.0 to 0.7;

start, primary display, table;

display and print semilog plot, minC 0.1, 4 cycles;

re-start same drug.


Change, sf(6) from 0.7 to 0.4;

start, primary display, table;

display and print semilog plot, minC 0.1, 4 cycles;

stop;

print results-log.
```

The results are shown as a series of semilog plots in *Figure 8.1*. The change of apparent plasma half-life with dose is shown by the change in slope of the plots.

Half-life and plasma concentrations increase as the hepatic function decreases; numerical values are shown in *Table 8.1*.

3.4 Plan for multi-dose regimens

The effect of hepatic function on steady-state plasma concentrations is examined in this set of runs.

Table 8.1 Paracetamol half-life, effect of hepatic dysfunction

Hepatic function	C at 1 h (mg/l)	$t_{1/2}$ (6–8 h) (h)
1.0	11.4	2.69
0.7	14.0	3.57
0.4	17.1	6.0

a

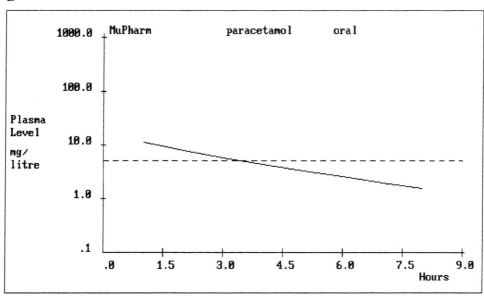

Press any key to continue

b

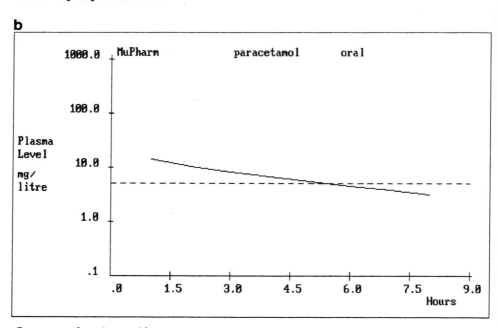

Press any key to continue

Figure 8.1 Paracetamol 1000 mg oral: **(a)** hepatic function = 1.0; **(b)** hepatic function = 0.7

c

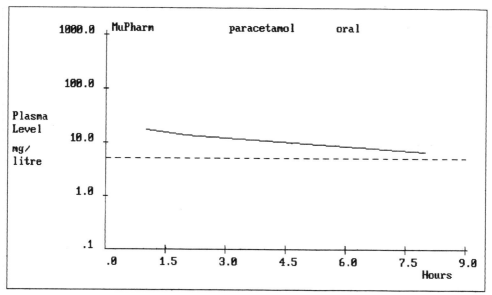

Press any key to continue

Figure 8.1 (c) hepatic function = 0.4

First, to assess the kinetic behaviour of paracetamol in the normal subject without hepatic dysfunction, three 12-h runs to determine area$_T$ are made at dose levels of 250, 1000 and 4000 mg oral. Since the apparent half-life at low doses is around 2.7 h, runs of 12 h are used.

Semilog plots of the results are made as before so that they can be compared as shown in *Figure 8.2*.

In view of the short half-life of paracetamol, a suitable dosing interval for a multi-dose regimen with the standard subject is 6 h.

The minimum active plasma level is 5 mg/l and the minimum toxic level is 120 mg/l (Appendix II); a target value of twice the active level, 10.0 mg/l, is used.

Assuming first-order kinetic behaviour in the first place, the dose required every 6 h to give the target mean steady-state value of C is estimated by equation (1.15), taking D_1 as 250 mg, the lowest dose used in the runs for area estimation.

$$D = D_1 \times C_{SS} \times I_D / \text{area}_T(D_1, \text{oral})$$

The dose is modified if required to give a satisfactory regimen for the standard subject. A change of hepatic function to 0.4 (a 60% loss of function) is made and a run is carried out with the same regimen. Finally the dose and interval are adjusted to give a satsfactory schedule for the patient with the hepatic dysfunction.

L. Saunders, D. Ingram and S. H. D. Jackson

3.5 **Runs and results**

3.5.1 *Area estimation*

The first three runs made to estimate the areas under the C,t curves following single doses of 250, 1000 and 4000 mg are set up consecutively, as outlined below.

```
Run details
```

```
Paracetamol 250mg oral;

run length 12h, 12 results, 0.25, 0.5, 0.75, 1, 1.25,
1.5, 2, 3, 4, 6, 8 and 12h;

standard subject;

start, primary display, table;

area estimation;

display and print semilog plot, minC 0.1, 4 cycles;

re-start same drug.
```

For the second run the prescription is altered to 1000 mg and the procedure is repeated.

```
Paracetamol 1000mg oral;

start, primary display, table;

area estimation;

display and print semilog plot, minC 0.1, 4 cycles;

re-start same drug.
```

For the third run the dose is changed to 4000 mg.

```
Paracetamol 4000mg oral;

start, primary display, table;

area estimation;

display and print semilog plot, minC 0.1, 4 cycles;
```

```
stop;
```

```
print results.log.
```

The C,t values from the three runs are shown in *Figure 8.2*. It is seen that the late time slopes of the 250- and 1000-mg plots are similar but the slope of the 4000-mg plot is shallower, indicating that at the highest dose there is distinct capacity-limited elimination.

In *Table 8.2*, areas, dose/area ratios (proportional to total clearances, $Cl_T = F \times D/\text{area}_T$) and 6- to 8-h apparent half-lives are given. The values in the last two columns show the saturation effect, dose/area decreases as the dose increases.

The medical consequences of the capacity-limited metabolism of paracetamol are less severe than those with phenytoin (Chapter 7, Section 4.2). The effect is less pronounced and the therapeutic ratio for paracetamol (120/5 = 24) is quite high, so that with normal dosing, toxic levels are unlikely to be reached.

3.5.2 *Multidose regimens*

Numerical values for equation (1.15) are taken from the area data from the run with a 250-mg dose; $\text{area}_T = 9.19$ h mg/l, the target C_{SS} has been chosen in the plan to be 10 mg/l and I_D is 6 h.

$$D = D_1 \times C_{SS} \times I_D/\text{area}_T(D_1,\text{oral}) = 250 \times 10.0 \times 6.0/9.19 = 1632 \text{ mg}$$

In view of the saturation effect, this value is rounded down to 1500 mg every 6 h.

A run of 48 h with peak, mid-interval and trough plasma concentrations is made, i.e. with results 1, 3 and 6 h after each dose. The run is set up as follows.

```
Run details
```

```
Paracetamol 1500mg every 6h for 8 doses, oral;
```

```
run length 48h, 24 results at 1, 3, 6, 7, 9, 12, 13, 15,
18, 19, 21, 24, 25, 27, 30, 31, 33, 36, 37, 39, 42, 43,
45, 48h;
```

```
standard subject;
```

```
start, primary display, table;
```

```
display and print semilog plot, auto minC and cycles;
```

```
restart same drug.
```

The semilog plot is shown in *Figure 8.3*. Apart from the trough at the end of the first dosing interval, the plasma concentrations are all well above the minimum active level.

a

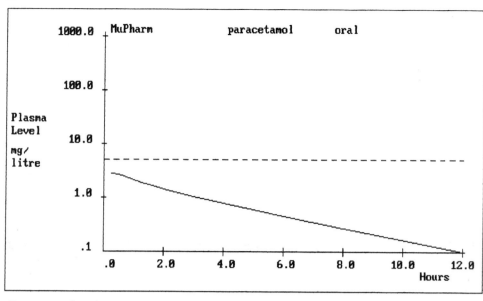

Press any key to continue

b

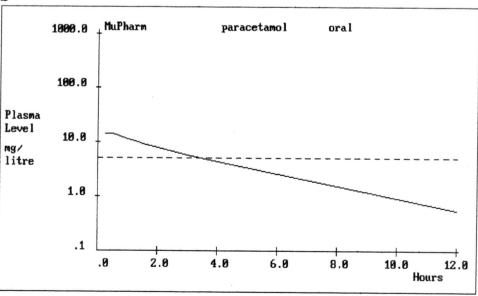

Press any key to continue

Figure 8.2 Paracetamol: (a) 250 mg oral; (b) 1000 mg oral

c

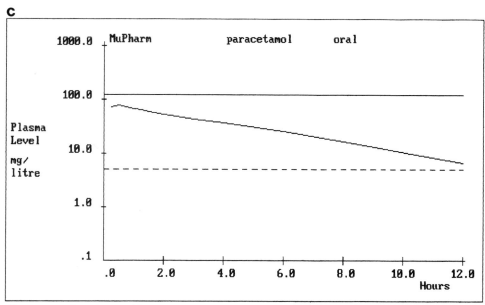

Press any key to continue
Figure 8.2 (c) 4000 mg oral.

Mid-interval values of C mg/l at times t are:

t (h)	3	9	15	21	27	33	39	45
C_{MI}	10.2	14.2	15.9	16.8	17.1	17.3	17.4	17.4

Table 8.2 Parameters for paracetamol

Dose (mg)	$area_T$ (h mg/l)	dose/$area_T$ (l/h)	$t_{1/2}$ (h)
250	9.19	27.2	2.64
1000	50.3	19.9	2.67
4000	395	10.1	3.15

The steady state is reached after the fifth dose with values of C_{MI} well above the target of 10 mg/l due to the capacity-limited effect. The dose could be reduced to give steady-state C_{MI} values closer to the target. If the dose is reduced in the proportion 10/17.4, it would be 867 mg; however, owing to the saturable metabolism effect, concentrations will not be directly proportional to doses and so a somewhat higher value of 1000 mg is used for the next run.

L. Saunders, D. Ingram and S. H. D. Jackson

```
Run details
```

```
Paracetamol 1000mg every 6h for 8 doses, oral;
```

```
start, primary display, table;
```

```
display and print semilog plot, auto minC and cycles;
```

```
restart same drug.
```

The semilog plot is shown in *Figure 8.4*. The troughs are now slightly below the minimum active level but the mean interval concentrations are closer to, though somewhat below, the target level.

t (h)	3	9	15	21	27	33	39	45
C_{MI}	5.7	7.6	8.3	8.5	8.6	8.6	8.6	8.6

This regimen is satisfactory.

3.5.3 Subject with a 60% loss of hepatic function

A 60% loss of hepatic function is given to the standard subject by reducing sf(6) to 0.4; the run is then repeated with the same dosage and timing schemes. At the end, a semilog plot is chosen and the results are shown in *Figure 8.5*.

```
Run details
```

```
Change, sf(6) from 1 to 0.4;
```

```
start, primary display, table;
```

```
display and print semilog plot, auto minC and cycles;
```

```
restart same drug.
```

It is seen that the C values are increasing over each dose interval; they are well below the toxic level but are far above the target mean steady-state concentration. The mid-interval C values in mg/l at times t are:

t (h)	3	9	15	21	27	33	39	45
C_{MI}	12.0	19.8	25.3	29.5	32.8	35.4	37.6	39.3

C_{MI} is increasing steadily and at 45 h it is almost four times the target.

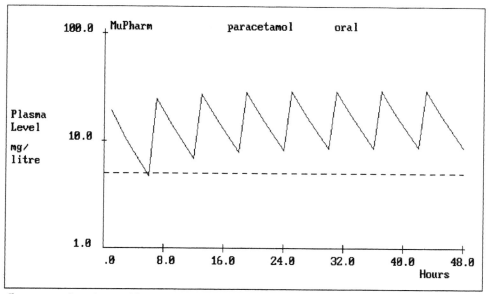

Press any key to continue

Figure 8.3 Paracetamol 1500 mg/6 h oral; hepatic function = 1.0.

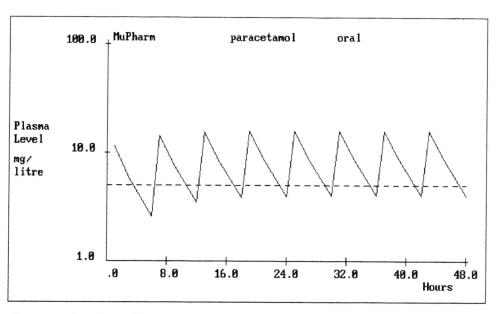

Press any key to continue

Figure 8.4 Paracetamol 1000 mg/6 h oral; hepatic function = 1.

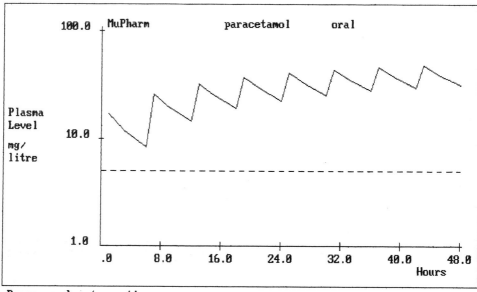

Press any key to continue

Figure 8.5 Paracetamol 1000 mg/6 h oral; hepatic function = 0.4.

A new run is made with a reduced dose of 500 mg and the same dosing interval of 6 h; eight doses are given with a run time of 48 h. The timings are the same. A semilog plot of the results is shown in *Figure 8.6* The subject is still the standard one with the hepatic dysfunction and does not have to be re-entered after restarting with the same drug.

```
Run details
```

```
Paracetamol 500mg every 6h for 8 doses, oral;

start, primary display, table;

display and print semilog plot, auto minC and cycles.
```

As the steady state is not reached at the end of the run, doses are continued for a further 48 h.

```
Run details
```

```
continue, with doses
```

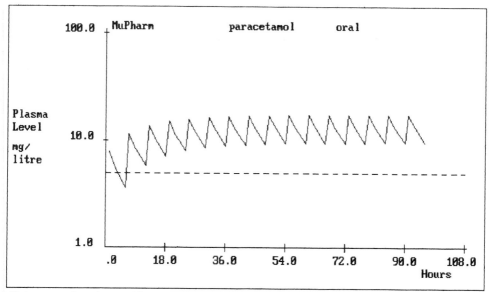

Press any key to continue

Figure 8.6 Paracetamol 500 mg/6 h; hepatic function = 0.4.

```
display and print semilog plot, automatic minC and
cycles.
```

The combined results are shown in *Figure 8.6*.

This regimen is satisfactory. The mid-interval C values in mg/l for the first run at times t are:

t (h)	3	9	15	21	27	33	39	45
C_{MI}	5.4	8.4	10.2	11.3	12.0	12.5	12.8	13.0

In the continued run, a steady state is reached after a total of 11 doses. The steady-state peak concentration, 17.4 mg/l, is well below the toxic level; the mid-interval level is 13.3; the trough value is 9.5, above the minimum active level. This regimen is therefore satisfactory for the patient with an hepatic dysfunction.

3.6 Conclusions

Hepatic dysfunctions result in increased plasma concentrations and half-lives, following single doses of paracetamol.

Paracetamol exhibits capacity-limited metabolism, the dose/area ratio decreasing as dose increases. A multidose regimen for the standard subject devised assuming first-order kinetics, gives an overestimate of the dose required. When an hepatic dysfunction is given to the subject, the plasma levels following repeated doses increase considerably. A reduced dose brings about a satisfactory steady state.

4. PARACETAMOL OVERDOSES

When an attempted suicide has involved the ingestion of large doses (many grams) of paracetamol, it is important to make an early assessment of possible permanent liver damage, so that treatment may be started as soon as possible. The standard treatment is now *N*-acetyl cysteine which enables the toxic metabolite to be further metabolized.

A graphical method which may be used for assessing liver damage following massive overdose is shown in *Figure 8.7* together with results generated from large doses of paracetamol in the simulation program, as described in experiment 13. In this method, two C,t points are plotted on semilog paper: the first is $C = 180$ mg/l at $t = 4$ h; the second is $C = 45$ mg/l at $t = 12$ h.

The two points are joined by a straight line and the patient's plasma level is determined at times 4, 8 and 12 h after the overdose. When the points representing these C,t values lie above the line, then serious liver damage is likely. This method combines half-life determination with the values of plasma concentration [L.F.Prescott, *Drugs*, (1983) **25**, 290–314].

5. EXPERIMENT 13: STUDIES WITH PARACETAMOL OVERDOSES

5.1 **Objective**

The simulation model may be used to examine overdose C,t data by giving a series of large doses to the standard subject and following the plasma concentrations. The objective is to test the concentration values obtained in order to determine whether treatment to counter possible liver damage should be started.

5.2 **Plan**

Doses of 5, 10, 15 and 20 g are used with runs of 12 h and four results at 4, 5, 8 and 12 h. Only the tables of results are required. The 5-h value is included so that an early assessment of the 4- to 5-h half- life may be made.

5.3 **Runs and results**

The runs are set up as follows.

```
Run details



Paracetamol 5000mg oral;

run length 12h, 4 results at 4, 5, 8 and 12h;

standard subject;

start, primary display, table;

restart same drug
```

```
Paracetamol 10000mg oral;

start, primary display, table;

restart same drug

Paracetamol 15000mg oral;

start, primary display, table;

restart same drug

Paracetamol 20000mg oral;

start, primary display, table;

stop;

print results-log.
```

The C,t values are given in *Table 8.3* and the 4-, 8- and 12-h C values are shown on a semilog plot together with the liver damage reference line in *Figure 8.7*.

Table 8.3 Plasma concentrations of paracetamol (mg/l) at times t following overdoses

Dose (g)	C (4 h)	C (5 h)	C (8 h)	C (12 h)	$t_{1/2}$ (4–5 h)
5	51.6	44.3	26.7	11.6	4.5
10	137	126	97.1	62.9	8.3
15	228	216	181	139	12.8
20	321	307	269	222	15.5

5.4 Conclusions

The 4- to 5-h half-lives provide the earliest warning of possible liver damage; values greater than 4 h have been taken to indicate that treatment should be started to counter possible liver damage. The values in the last column of *Table 8.3* suggest that treatment should be started in all cases.

The indications from *Figure 8.7* are that the 5-g dose plot is well below the reference line and so liver damage is not to be expected; the 10-g dose plot crosses the line and the 15- and 20-g dose results are well above the reference line. In these three cases, liver damage is probable. The determination of the 4- to 5-h half-life alone may produce false positive assessments of the need for treatment, as with the 5-g dose above.

167

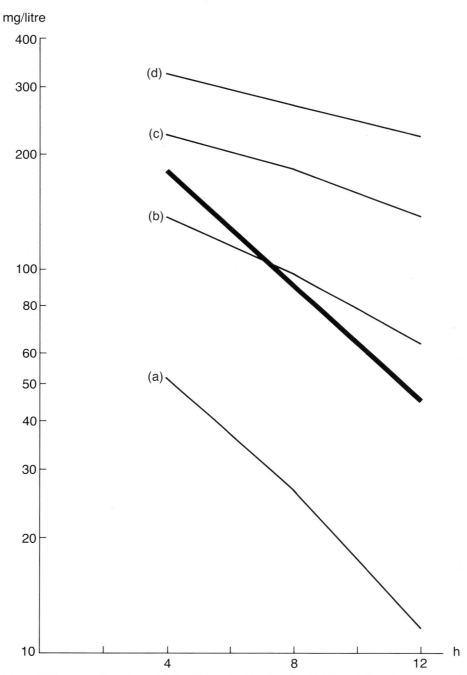

Figure 8.7 Paracetamol overdoses: (a) 5 g; (b) 10 g; (c) 15 g; (d) 20 g. (Thick line is liver damage reference line.)

6. EXPERIMENT 14: TO STUDY THE EFFECTS OF RENAL IMPAIRMENT ON THE PHARMACOKINETICS OF GENTAMICIN

6.1 Objective

The objective is to devise a multidose schedule for the standard subject with gentamicin given by the i.m. route. The effect of renal impairment in the subject is then examined and a new schedule is developed.

6.2 Plan

6.2.1 *Effect of renal impairment on gentamicin dosing*

Renal impairment affects the plasma levels of drugs which are mainly eliminated unchanged in the urine. Many antibiotics are in this category and gentamicin (Chapter 3, Section 4) is taken as an example. The minimum active plasma level for gentamicin is 4 mg/l and the toxic level is 12 mg/l (Appendix II).

The area under the C,t curve, with a single i.m. dose of 120 mg of gentamicin given to the standard subject, has been determined in Chapter 3, Section 4.3 as 27.9 mg h/l.

The recommendation for repeated dosing with gentamicin is that at the steady state, the peak concentration should be above 8 mg/l but below the toxic level, and the steady-state trough concentration should be between 1 and 3 mg/l. This second requirement means that the troughs will be below the minimum active level.

The half-life is quite short, 2.5 h, and so the dosing interval is set at 6 h; a steady-state target level of 6 mg/l is used.

Gentamicin exhibits first-order elimination and the repeated dose for this regimen is calculated from equation (1.15).

$$D = D_1 \times C_{SS} \times I_D / \text{area}_T (D_1, \text{i.m.}) = 120 \times 6 \times 6/27.9 = 155 \text{ mg}$$

A repeated-dose run is set up with a dose of 150 mg i.m. of gentamicin, every 6 h for four doses, with results at the peak concentration (1 h after dose), the mid-point (3 h after dose) and the trough (6 h after dose); a table is chosen for the primary display and a semilog plot is chosen for the final display of results.

6.3 Runs and results

The runs are set up as described below.

```
Run details



Gentamicin, 150mg every 6h for 4 doses, IM;

run length 24h; 12 results at 1, 3, 6, 7, 9, 12, 13, 15,
18, 19, 21, 24h;
```

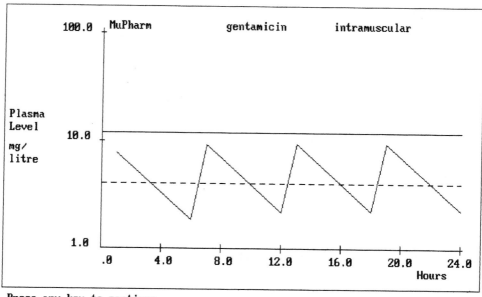

Press any key to continue

Figure 8.8 Gentamicin 150 mg/6 h i.m.; *GFR* = 7.5 l/h.

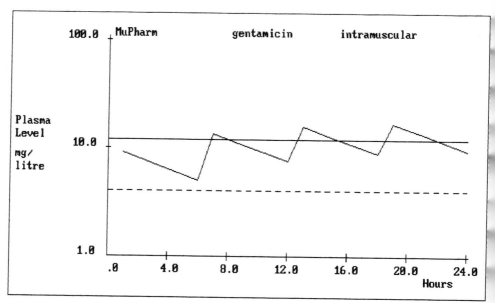

Press any key to continue

Figure 8.9 Gentamicin 150 mg/6 h i.m.; *GFR* = 3 l/h.

170

```
standard subject;

start, primary display, table;

display and print semilog plot, automatic minC and
cycles;

restart same drug.
```

The semilog plot is shown in *Figure 8.8*. Plasma concentrations are above the minimum active level for 60% of the later dosing intervals.

The values of plasma concentration in mg/l are:

Dose	1	2	3	4
Peak	7.7	9.1	9.4	9.4
C_{MI}	4.4	5.2	5.3	5.3
Trough	1.8	2.2	2.2	2.3

These results comply with the requirements for peak and trough values, and give a satisfactory regimen for the standard subject.

6.3.1 *Patient with renal impairment*

The next run is made with the same regimen as the previous one but with the standard subject given a 60% loss of renal function. This loss of function is set by altering the glomerular filtration rate (*GFR*, subject factor 9) from the normal value of 7.5 l/h for the standard subject, to $0.4 \times 7.5 = 3$ l/h.

After restarting with the same drug, subject factor 9 is altered to 3 l/h. The dose, timings and primary display are left unchanged; at the end of the run a semilog plot is chosen.

```
Run details



Change, sf(9) from 7.5 to 3.0;

Start, primary display, table;

display and print semilog plot, auto minC and cycles;

restart same drug.
```

The semilog plot is shown in *Figure 8.9*.

The peak, mid-interval and trough plasma concentrations C in mg/l are:

Dose	1	2	3	4
Peak	9.0	13.5	15.7	16.9
C_{MI}	7.1	10.7	12.5	13.3
Trough	5.0	7.5	8.8	9.4

The half-life of the drug is considerably increased by the dysfunction; an estimate of this half-life from the 3- and 6-h results is 5.9 h. Toxic levels are reached after the second dose and the last mid-interval C value is more than twice the target value, with no sign of a steady state.

Clearly the regimen would be unsuitable for this patient — the toxic effects of gentamicin include renal damage and the possibility of permanent deafness. A satisfactory regimen is devised below.

6.3.2 Regimen for the patient with renal impairment

The 150-mg dose every 6 h is too high; in view of the more than doubled half-life, the dosing interval could be doubled. For a new regimen, the dose is reduced to 120 mg and the dosing interval is increased to 12 h. The timings need to be changed to fit this new interval. After restart same drug, the change in *GFR* does not have to be re-entered.

The next run is made with this regimen.

```
Run details



Gentamicin 120mg every 12h for 4 doses IM;

run length 48h, 12 results, 1, 6, 12, 13, 18, 24, 25, 30,
36, 37, 42, 48h;
```

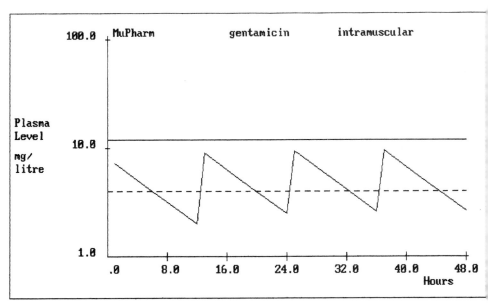

```
Press any key to continue
```
Figure 8.10 Gentamicin 120 mg/12 h i.m.; *GFR* = 3 l/h.

```
start, primary display, table;

display and print semilog plot, auto minC and cycles;

restart same drug
```

The semilog plot is shown in *Figure 8.10.*

Plasma levels are in the active range for 64% of the later intervals and a steady state is reached with peak and trough plasma concentrations in the correct ranges.

The peak, mid-interval and trough plasma concentration values in mg/l are:

Dose	1	2	3	4
Peak	7.2	9.0	9.4	9.6
C_{MI}	4.0	5.0	5.3	5.3
Trough	2.0	2.5	2.6	2.7

The peak values are well below the toxic level and the regimen is satisfactory for this subject.

6.4 Conclusions

When an i.m. dose regimen suitable for the standard subject is given to a subject with a 60% loss of renal function, plasma levels rise rapidly into the toxic region and the half-life is more than doubled. A satisfactory regimen for this patient is developed by doubling the dosing interval and reducing the dose.

One of the possible toxic effects of gentamicin is renal impairment. If such a dysfunction occurs during the course of treatment with gentamicin, further serious toxicity may result.

7. PROBLEMS

1. Compare the effects of loss of renal and hepatic functions respectively, on oral dose regimens with the two beta-blockers, oxprenolol and atenolol.
2. Using some of the other drugs available, carry out simulation studies similar to those described in this chapter. In addition to the subject factors controlling hepatic and renal function, other subject and drug factors may be varied, e.g. drug factor 7 to modify protein binding, subject factor 2 to simulate change in cardiac output, subject factor 7 to simulate diuresis.
   Complete lists of the factors are given in Appendices III and IV.

CHAPTER 9

Doses, Responses and Regimens with Different Subjects. Studies with Temazepam, Paracetamol, Phenytoin and Digoxin

1. INTRODUCTION

In this chapter the responses of different subjects to some drugs are compared. Up to this point in the book the examples have all used the standard simulation model subject, a 25-year-old male of body mass 70 kg and height 183 cm.

A different subject may be chosen in the program by specifying the height, weight, age and sex of this new subject. The relevant subject factors (see Appendix III) are calculated automatically to give values appropriate to such a subject. Further adjustment of individual factors such as hepatic function or glomerular filtration rate may then be made, so as to describe particular patients.

2. EXPERIMENT 15: TO COMPARE THE EFFECTS OF TEMAZEPAM ON TWO SUBJECTS

2.1 Objective

Temazepam is a short-acting metabolite of diazepam and is used to induce sleep and to give sedation before surgical operations.

The objective of the experiment is to compare the plasma concentrations of the drug from single doses found with an elderly female, and with the standard subject.

2.2 Plan

The minimum plasma level of temazepam for activity is taken as 0.3 mg/l in the simulation.

A suitable dose for an old lady is 10 mg. This dose is given orally to a female subject (age 80 years, weight 50 kg and height 137 cm) in the simulation model. As a short-term response is required to induce sleep, the run is made for 9 h with results every half hour.

The same dose is then given to the standard subject and is revised so as to give a concentration–time curve similar to that for the elderly subject.

2.3 Runs and results

The run with the elderly subject is set up below.

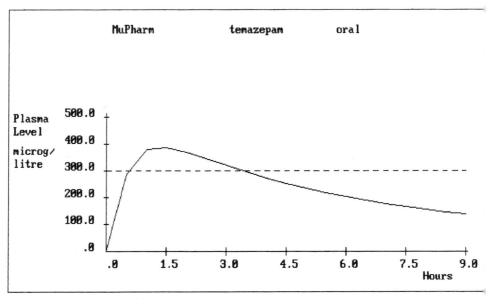

Press any key to continue
Figure 9.1 Temazepam 10 mg oral, 80-year-old female.

Run details

Temazepam 10mg oral;

run length 9h, 18 results, at 0.5h intervals;

subject, height 137, mass 50, age 80, female;

start, primary display, graph;

display and print C,t plot;

restart same drug.

The C,t plot is shown in *Figure 9.1*. The C,t curve is above the broken horizontal line from
0.5 h to 3.2 h, which should be sufficient for inducing sleep.
The same dose is given to the standard subject.

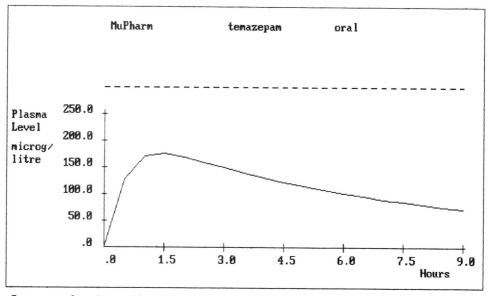

Press any key to continue
Figure 9.2 Temazepam 10 mg oral, standard subject.

```
Run details



subject, standard;

start, primary display, graph;

display and print C,t plot;

restart same drug.
```

Figure 9.2 shows the *C,t* plot. The plasma concentrations are all below the broken line. Temazepam shows first-order kinetics so that plasma concentrations are proportional to dose. By inspection of the two figures, it is seen that a doubling of the dose to 20 mg for the standard subject should give plasma concentrations with the standard subject similar to those with the elderly female. A run with this dose is set up below.

```
Run details



Temazepam 20mg oral;
```

```
start, primary display, graph;

display and print C,t plot;

stop.
```

Figure 9.3 displays the *C,t* values. There is now a period during which the curve is above the broken line from 0.7 h to 3 h, similar to that obtained with the first subject.

2.4 Conclusions

These results show that in order to obtain similar plasma concentrations of temazepam with the standard subject as with the elderly lady, the dose needs to be doubled.

3. EXPERIMENT 16: TO DEVELOP A SUITABLE REGIMEN FOR PARACETAMOL WITH A YOUNG CHILD

3.1 Objective

Paracetamol is used for treating mild pain and is often given to children. It has a high therapeutic index and therefore does not present a hazard unless substantial overdoses are taken, when liver damage can occur (Chapter 8, Section 2).

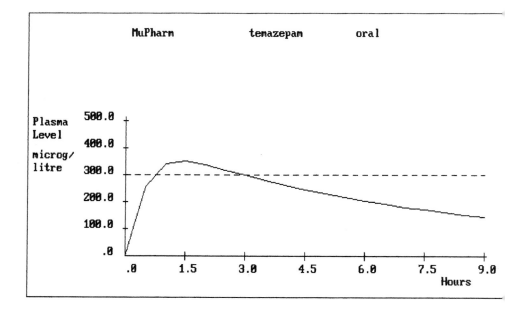

Press any key to continue

Figure 9.3 Temazepam 20 mg oral, standard subject.

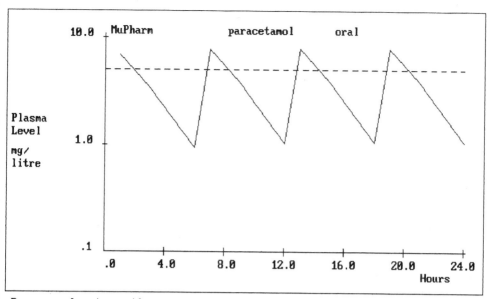

Press any key to continue

Figure 9.4 Paracetamol 120 mg/6 h, 1-year-old boy, scaled by body mass.

The objective of this experiment is to develop a paracetamol regimen suitable for a male child aged 1 year.

3.2 Plan

In Chapter 8, Section 3.5, a satisfactory regimen for paracetamol with the standard subject, a 25-year-old male of mass 70 kg, has been evaluated as 1000 mg/6 h. A regimen is now developed for a boy of age 1 year, mass 8.5 kg and height 75 cm.

In the first place, the dose for the child is calculated by simple scaling of the masses of the two subjects:

$$D = 8.5/70 \times 1000 = 121 \text{ mg}$$

This dose is rounded to 120 mg every 6 h. A 24-h run is made with peak, mid-interval and trough concentration results; the primary display is the table and a semilog plot is finally displayed. The preference for a semilog plot for results of multi-dose runs has been discussed in Chapter 6, Section 6.3.

3.3 Runs and results

The first run is set up as described below.

```
Run details
```

```
Paracetamol 120mg every 6h for 4 doses oral;
```

```
run length 24h with 12 results at times 1, 3, 6, 7, 9,
12, 13, 15, 18, 19, 21, 24h;
```

```
subject, 75cm, 8.5kg, 1y, male;
```

```
start, primary display, table;
```

```
display and print semilog plot, auto minC and cycles;
```

```
restart same drug.
```

The C,t values are shown in *Figure 9.4*. It is seen that most of the plot is below the active level. The time for which concentration values are effective is estimated by measuring within a dose interval the times at which the plot is above and below the minimum active level indicated by the broken horizontal line.

For the fourth dose in *Figure 9.4* these times are, active 1.6 h, inactive 4.4 h. The drug is therefore only active for 26% of the time — an unsatisfactory result.

Particularly for children, it is found that dose scaling should be done on a basis of body area rather than body mass. The two ratios do not differ greatly for older children (>12 years) and adults, but for very young children the area ratio is substantially larger than the mass ratio.

The values of total body surface area for a subject are calculated from height and body mass by a venerable formula proposed by Dubois and Dubois in 1916 [*Arch. Intern. Med.* (1916) **17**, 863, see Martindale]:

$$\text{Area} = W^{0.425} \times H^{0.725} \times 71.84/10\,000 \text{ m}^2$$

(9.1)

where W is mass in kg and H is height in cm.

Using this formula, the area for the standard subject is 1.91 m^2, while that for the young boy is 0.408 m^2, giving an area ratio of 0.214, substantially larger than the mass ratio of 0.121.

The dose of paracetamol scaled by the surface area ratio is 214 mg, which is rounded to 220 mg every 6 h for the next run with the 1-year-old boy.

```
Run details
```

```
Paracetamol 220mg every 6h for 4 doses oral;
```

```
start, primary display, table;

display and print semilog plot, auto minC and cycles;

restart same drug.
```

The *C,t* results are shown in *Figure 9.5*. The active plasma levels are now obtained for 4.4 h of the 6-h dosing interval, i.e. for 74% of the time; the dose could be further increased to 250mg.

3.4 Conclusions

In general, small children eliminate drugs more rapidly than would be expected from their mass ratio to an adult, consequently the use of the mass ratio to scale child to adult doses results in underdoses; the body surface area ratio should be used.

These scaling processes may not be reliable for drugs which show substantial capacity-limited effects in the therapeutic dose range; with paracetamol this effect is present but is not substantial at concentrations near the minimum active level.

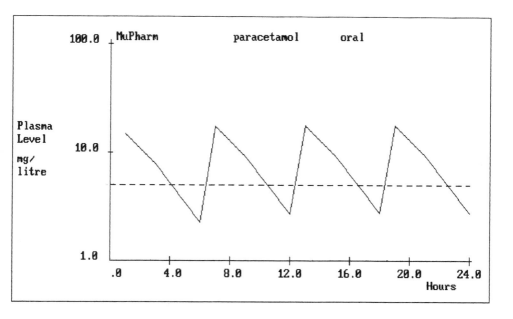

Press any key to continue

Figure 9.5 Paracetamol 220 mg /6 h oral, 1-year-old subject, scaled by area.

4. EXPERIMENT 17: TO DEVELOP A REGIMEN FOR TREATMENT OF A CHILD WITH PHENYTOIN

4.1 Objective

Phenytoin has been described in Chapter 7. The low therapeutic index (C_{act} = 10 and C_{tox} = 20 mg/l) and the capacity-limited kinetic behaviour mean that great care has to be taken in designing dosage schemes with children.

The objective of this experiment is to devise a phenytoin regimen suitable for a 6-year-old boy of height 118 cm and body mass 22 kg. First a run is made with the adult dose given to this child.

4.2 Plan for adult dose

A run is first made with the boy subject, using the dosing schedule designed for the standard subject in Chapter 7, Section 4.8, 300 mg/24 h with a loading dose of 700 mg. A run length of 144 h is used with peak, mid-interval and trough values of plasma concentration.

4.3 Run and results: adult dose

The adult dose is given in the run set out below.

```
Run details
```

```
Phenytoin 300mg every 24h for 6 doses oral, loading dose
700mg in 2 portions at 12h intervals;

run length 144h with 12 results at 4, 24, 28, 48, 52, 72,
76, 96, 100, 120, 124, 144h;

subject, 118cm, 22kg, 6y, male;

start, primary display, graph;

display and print semilog plot, auto minC and cycles;

restart same drug.
```

The primary display graph is shown in *Figure 9.6*. The results are disastrous with plasma concentration reaching the toxic level (denoted by the full horizontal line in the figure) after a few hours. The concentration continues to increase until the run is terminated after the 48-h dose because, unhappily, the simulated subject dies of phenytoin poisoning.

When the subject dies, the execution of the program stops and a further plot cannot be made. You are returned to the CONTROL menu where a new dose has to be prescribed and a new subject has to be selected.

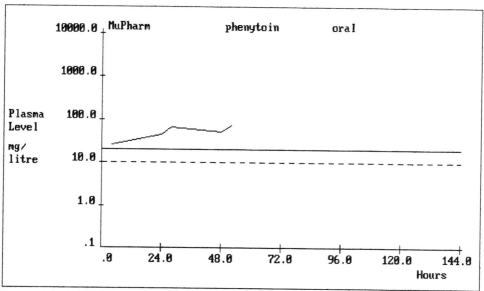

Your subject has died of an overdose; reset subject and prescription

Figure 9.6 Phenytoin 700 + 300 mg/24 h, 6-year-old boy.

4.4 Evaluation of appropriate child doses

4.4.1 *Loading dose*

Some 24-h simulation runs similar to those in Chapter 7, Section 4.5, are made starting with safe low doses, to establish a suitable loading dose for the boy subject. A dose of 225 mg in three divided portions at 8-h intervals is found to give a 24-h plasma concentration in the active region without approaching the toxic level.

The 24-h run with this dose is set up as described below.

```
Run details


Phenytoin 75mg every 8h for 3 doses oral;

run length 24h, 24 results every 1h;

subject, 118cm, 22kg, 6y, male;

start, primary display, table;

display and print semilog plot, auto minC and cycles;
```

```
restart same drug.
```

Because the previous subject died, the characteristics of the new subject, which are the same, have to be re-entered. The semilog plot is shown in *Figure 9.7*.

4.4.2 *Maintenance dose*

The size of the maintenance dose to be used with the 225-mg loading dose is explored next. Direct scaling of the adult dose of 300 mg by the mass ratio 22/70 gives 94 mg.

The body surface area of the child subject, calculated using equation (9.1), is 0.85 m^2 and the maintenance dose scaled by area is 0.85/1.91 × 300 = 134 mg.

Direct scaling with a drug exhibiting saturable metabolism may not be reliable and a third estimate is made by using the Michaelis–Menten equation with an estimated V_{max} value for the boy.

In Chapter 7, Section 3.4 values of the capacity-limited elimination phenytoin parameters for the standard subject have been calculated as K_m = 8.23 mg/l, V_{max} = 18.0 mg/h.

K_m is likely to have similar values for a range of subjects, while V_{max} should be scaled, preferably by the area ratio. The estimate of V_{max} for the boy is therefore 18.0 × 0.85/1.91 = 8.0 mg/h.

With these parameters, the maintenance dose may be estimated using equation (7.1).

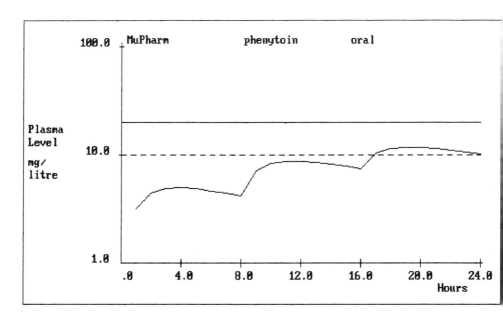

Press any key to continue

Figure 9.7 Phenytoin 75 mg/8 h oral, 6-year-old boy.

The assumptions made are that the renal excretion of unchanged drug is negligible and that the drug is completely absorbed from an oral dose, both of which are approximately true for phenytoin. The argument for estimating a maintenance dose is similar to that used in Chapter 7, Section 4.6, leading to equation (9.2) below.

$$D = I_D \times V_{max} \times C_{MI}/(K_m + C_{MI})$$

(9.2)

Substituting numerical values into this equation with a target value of 15 mg/l for C_{MI} gives:

$$D = 24 \times 8.0 \times 15/(8.23 + 15) = 124 \text{ mg}$$

This and the other two estimates indicate that an appropriate maintenance dose for the boy is likely to be between 100 and 150 mg/24 h and so a run is made with the loading dose plus a maintenance dose at the bottom of this range: 100 mg/24 h.

4.5 Runs and results: maintenance dose

The timings for the run are as in Section 4.3, but need to be re-entered.

```
Run details
```

```
Phenytoin 100mg every 24h for 6 doses oral, loading dose
225mg in 3 portions at 8h intervals;

run length 144h with 18 results at 4, 12, 24, 28, 36, 48,
52, 60, 72, 76, 84, 96, 100, 108, 120, 124, 132, 144h;

start, primary display, table;
```

The mid-interval plasma concentrations in mg/l are shown below.

t (h)	12	36	60	84	108	132
C_{MI}	8.7	12.7	10.4	8.9	8.1	7.6

In order to determine the steady-state concentration, the run is continued for a further 144 h with the doses repeated.

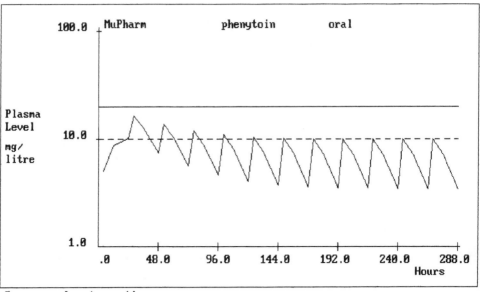

Press any key to continue

Figure 9.8 Phenytoin 225 mg + 100mg/24 h, 6-year-old boy.

Run details

Continue with doses;

display and print semilog plot, auto minC and cycles;

restart same drug.

The mid-interval C values in mg/l are:

t (h)	156	180	204	228	252	276
C_{MI}	7.4	7.2	7.2	7.2	7.1	7.1

The semilog plot of the run and its continuation are shown in *Figure 9.8*.

The results above show that the steady state is closely approached after the 10th dose. In general, with capacity-limited kinetics, it takes a long time for a steady state to be established.

This maintenance dose is clearly too low, allowing the plasma concentrations to fall below the active level. In the next run, this dose is increased to 150 mg. It is only necessary to alter the prescription from the previous run.

186

Run details

Phenytoin, 150mg every 24h for 6 doses oral, loading dose
225mg in 3 portions at 8h intervals;.

start, primary display, table;

The mid-interval *C* results are:

t (h)	12	36	60	84	108	132
C_{MI}	8.7	16.6	16.9	17.1	17.3	17.4

The run is continued for a further 144 h with doses.

t (h)	156	180	204	228	252	276
CMI	17.5	17.6	17.6	17.7	17.7	17.7

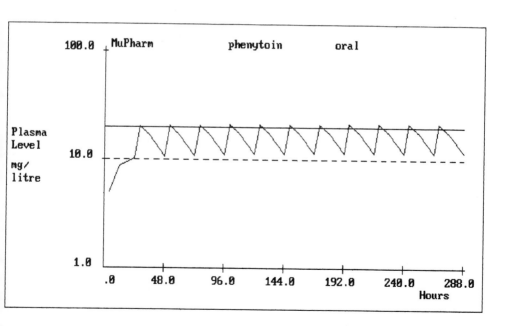

Press any key to continue

Figure 9.9 Phenytoin 150 mg/24 h, 6-year-old boy.

187

The combined results are shown as a semilog plot in *Figure 9.9* where it is seen that the peak values are in the toxic range.

4.6 Interpolation of maintenance dose using the Michaelis–Menten equation

The maintenance dose of 150 mg is too high. An approximate interpolation between the 100-mg and 150-mg doses may be made by using equation (9.2), based on the Michaelis–Menten equation.

The assumptions made in this interpolation are those for equation (9.2), namely that the renal excretion of unchanged drug is negligible and that the drug is completely absorbed from an oral dose.

If C_1 and C_2 mg/l are the steady-state concentrations at two dosing levels D_1 and D_2 mg, then substituting these two pairs of values D_2,C_2 and D_1,C_1 into equation (9.2):

$$D_2 = I_D \times V_{max} \times C_2/(K_m + C_2)$$

$$D_1 = I_D \times V_{max} \times C_1/(K_m + C_1)$$

Dividing the upper equation by the lower one

$$D_2/D_1 = C_2(K_m + C_1)/[C_1(K_m + C_2)]$$

Substituting the numerical values $D_2 = 150, D_1 = 100, C_2 = 17.7, C_1 = 7.1$ gives $K_m = 8.93$ mg/l.

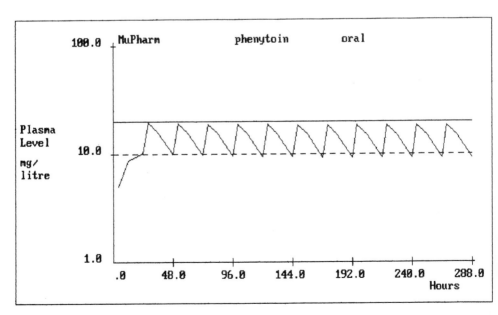

Press any key to continue

Figure 9.10 Phenytoin 225 mg + 140 mg/h oral, 6-year-old boy.

To calculate a value of V_{max} the larger dose values are used:

$$V_{max} = D_2 \times (K_m + C_2)/(I_D \times C_2)$$
$$V_{max} = 150 \times (8.93 + 17.7)/(24 \times 17.7) = 9.40 \text{ mg/h}$$

These values of K_m and V_{max} are in moderate agreement with the estimates $K_m = 8.23$ mg/l and $V_{max} = 8.0$ mg/h used in Section 4.4.

The maintenance dose required to give the target of 15 mg/l for C_{MI} is from equation (9.2):

$$D = I_D \times V_{max} \times C_{MI}/(K_m + C_{MI})$$

$$D = 24 \times 9.4 \times 15/(8.93 + 15) = 141 \text{ mg}$$

This value is rounded to 140 mg every 24 h and the next run is made with this maintenance dose.

```
Run details
```

```
Phenytoin,  140mg  every  24h  for  6  doses  oral,  loading  dose
225mg  in  3  portions  at  8h  intervals;
```

```
start,  primary  display,  table;
```

The results up to 144 h appear to be satisfactory and so the run is continued to 288 h.

```
Run details
```

```
Continue  with  doses
```

```
display  and  print  semilog  plot,  auto  minC  and  cycles;
```

```
stop.
```

The semilog plot continued up to 288 h is shown in *Figure 9.10*; the steady state is reached with peak concentrations below the toxic level. The trough concentrations do dip just below the active level; however, the proportion of a dosing interval for which plasma concentrations are below the active level is small.

4.7 Conclusions

After a disastrous run in which the 6-year-old child was given an adult dose of phenytoin, runs to evaluate a suitable loading dose have been made. A suitable maintenance dose has been estimated by several methods and tested cautiously, so as to give steady-state mean plasma concentrations at two doses.

Values of the Michaelis–Menten parameters are assessed from these results and are then used to interpolate between these two doses, to give a suitable regimen for the 6-year-old boy.

5. EXPERIMENT 18: TO EVALUATE REGIMENS FOR DIGOXIN WITH THE STANDARD SUBJECT, WITH A SMALL CHILD AND WITH AN ELDERLY SUBJECT

5.1 Objective

Digoxin is used to slow the heart rate in patients with cardiac failure. It is a potent drug with a fraction of a milligram as a normal dose; the therapeutic index is relatively small, the minimum active plasma concentration is 1 µg/l and the toxic level is 3 µg/l.

The objectives are to devise a multiple dosing schedule for oral digoxin with the standard subject, then with a 1.5-year-old boy and then with an 80-year-old man.

5.2 Plan

Since the kinetic behaviour of digoxin is first-order, scaling methods are used to adjust doses.

A single-dose run to estimate area under the curve for the standard subject is first made. The half-life of digoxin is 40 h, so a run length of 120 h is used with suitable timings. The dose is 0.4 mg oral.

Some 24-h runs are made to evaluate a suitable loading dose which will give rapid and continuing active levels. From the area results a maintenance dose is estimated and the schedule is tested by setting up a 144-h run in the first place, with peak, mid-interval and trough concentration values; the results are displayed on a semilog plot.

The standard subject doses are then scaled for the 1.5-year-old, first by the mass ratio and then by the body surface area ratio. The same runs are used and the results displayed on semilog plots.

The regimen for the standard subject is applied to the 80-year-old of the same body mass and height, different plasma concentrations due to the age effect are noted and a new schedule is designed for this subject.

5.3 Runs and results

5.3.1 *Digoxin regimen for the standard subject*

The first run, to determine the area under the curve with a single dose of digoxin, is made with the run set out below.

```
Run Details
```

```
Digoxin 0.4mg oral;
```

```
run length 120h, 19 results at 0.25, 0.5, 0.75, 1, 1.25,
1.5, 2, 3, 4, 6, 8, 12, 18, 24, 36, 48, 72, 96 and 120h;
```

```
standard subject;

start, primary display, graph;

area estimation;

restart same drug.
```

From the area estimation, the half-life is 42.1 h and the total area under the *C,t* plot is 46.6 h µg/l or 0.0466 h mg/l.

In view of the long half-life, a dosing interval of 24 h is chosen, the target steady-state mean concentration is taken between active and toxic levels 1.5 µg/l or 0.0015 mg/l. The maintenance dose is then estimated from equation (1.15);

$$D = D_1 \times C_{SS} \times I_D/\text{area}_T(D_1,\text{oral})$$

$$D = 0.4 \times 0.0015 \times 24/0.0466 = 0.31 \text{ mg}$$

This value is rounded to 0.3 mg/24 h.

Because of the half-life, it will take a long time for the steady-state plasma concentration to be reached. A loading dose will therefore be required if early action of the drug is necessary.

A series of 24 h runs are made to evaluate a loading dose which gives active levels rapidly and which results in a plasma concentration near to and above the active level at 24 h. These studies indicate that a loading dose of 0.75 mg given in three portions at 8-h intervals is appropriate.

The 144-h run with this schedule, 0.75 + 0.3 mg/24 h, is set up below.

```
Run Details
```

```
Digoxin 0.3mg every 24h for 6 doses, oral, loading dose
0.75mg in 3 portions at 8h intervals;

run length 144h, 18 results at 1, 12, 24, 25, 36, 48, 49,
60, 72, 73, 84, 96, 97, 108, 120, 121, 132, 144h;

start, primary display, graph;

display and print semilog plot, minC = 0.1, 2 cycles;

restart same drug.
```

The minimum concentration and number of cycles are specified, because the automatic choice makes the time axis coincide with and obscure the broken line indicating the active level.

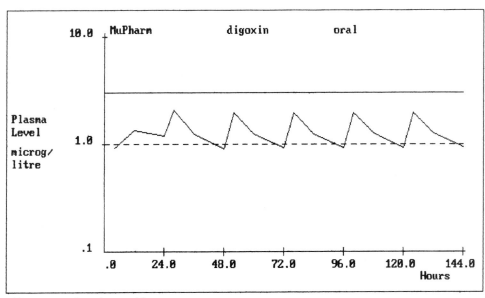

Press any key to continue

Figure 9.11 Digoxin 0.75 + 0.3 mg//24 h, standard subject.

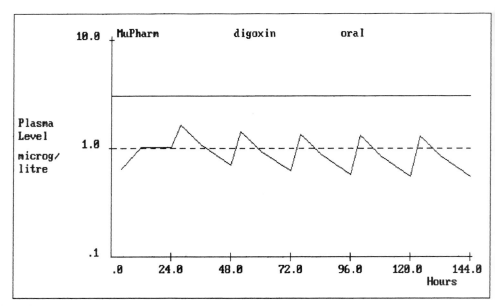

Press any key to continue

Figure 9.12 Digoxin 0.12 + 0.05 mg/24 h, 1.5-year-old boy.

The results are shown in *Figure 9.11* and it is seen that the regimen is satisfactory, with a slight dip below the active level at the end of each interval.

5.3.2 *Digoxin regimen for 1.5-year-old boy*

The child subject for the next run is a 1.5-year-old boy of body mass 11.4 kg and height 82 cm. The doses are scaled to those for the standard subject by the mass ratio 11.5/70 = 0.162, resulting in a loading dose of 0.12 mg in three portions and a maintenance dose of 0.05 mg every 24 h.

The run to test this regimen is set up below; the run timings do not have to be re-entered after the restart.

```
Run details
```

```
Digoxin 0.05mg every 24h for 6 doses oral,loading dose
0.12mg in 3 portions at 8h intervals;

subject, 82cm, 11.4kg, 1.5y, male;

primary display, graph;

display and print semilog plot, minC = 0.1, cycles = 2;

restart same drug.
```

The results shown in *Figure 9.12* are unsatisfactory because the plasma levels are below the minimum active level for 15 h in the last dosing interval of 24 h, i.e. for 63% of the time.

As with paracetamol (Section 3.3), the answer is to use the area ratio for scaling. The Dubois equation gives the body area for this subject as:

$$\text{body surface area} = 11.4^{0.425} \times 82^{0.725} \times 71.84/10\,000$$

$$= 2.813 \times 24.41 \times 71.84/10\,000$$

$$= 0.493 \text{ m}^2$$

The body surface area of the standard subject is 1.91 m^2 and the scaling ratio is therefore 0.493/1.91 = 0.258. The maintenance dose is then estimated from that for the standard subject as 0.08 mg every 24 h; the loading dose in the previous run was satisfactory and so is kept at 0.12 mg in three portions.

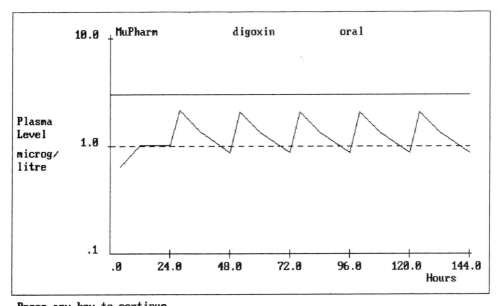

Press any key to continue

Figure 9.13 Digoxin 0.12 + 0.08 mg/24 h, 1.5-year-old boy.

Run details

Digoxin 0.08mg every 24h for 6 doses oral, loading dose
0.12mg in 3 portions at 8h intervals;

start, primary display, graph;

display and print semilog plot, minC = 0.1, cycles = 2;

restart same drug.

The results are shown in *Figure 9.13* and are now satisfactory.

5.3.3 *Digoxin regimen with 80-year-old subject*

Advancing years generally cause a reduction in body weight and in body fluid volume so
that the volume of distribution is reduced. An old man of 80 years given drug doses
developed for a 25-year-old shows higher plasma levels. However, the ratio of steady-
state plasma concentrations (80-year-old)/(25-year-old) is often more than would be
expected from the ratio of distribution volumes.

With drugs showing first-order kinetic behaviour this effect is mainly due to reduced
renal function for the elderly subject, with some contribution from reduced hepatic

194

function. With drugs which show saturable metabolism the effect is also partly due to increased saturation of liver enzymes.

In this study an 80-year-old male is used, with the same height (183 cm) and body mass (70 kg) as the standard subject so that the differences in plasma concentrations are due solely to the effects of age.

In the first run, the regimen for the standard subject, 0.75 + 0.3 mg/24 h is repeated with the 80-year-old.

```
Run details



Digoxin 0.3mg every 24h for 6 doses oral, loading dose
0.75mg in 3 portions at 8h intervals;

subject, 183cm, 70kg, 80y, male;

start, primary display, graph;

display and print semilog plot, minC = 0.1, cycles = 2;

restart same drug.
```

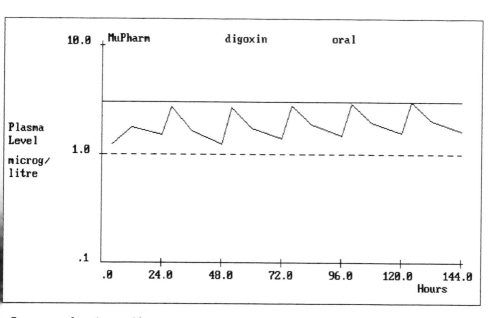

Press any key to continue

Figure 9.14 Digoxin 0.75 + 0.3 mg/h oral, 80-year-old subject.

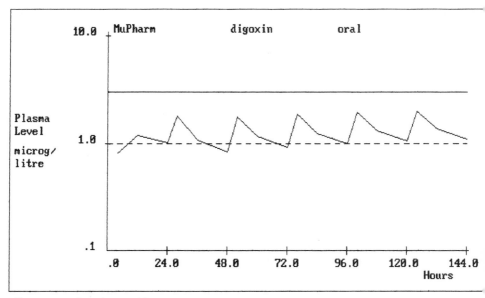

Figure 9.15 Digoxin 0.5 + 0.2 mg/h oral, 80-year-old subject.

The results in *Figure 9.14* show that at 120 h the peak concentration is in the toxic range, the plasma levels are increasing and so continuing toxicity is to be expected.

The reason for this result can be found by making a 120-h single-dose run to determine half-life when this subject receives 0.3 mg of digoxin. The late time $t_{1/2}$ is found to be 72.6 h compared with 42.1 h for the standard subject.

The doses are adjusted to give a more acceptable regimen for the 80-year-old by scaling down according to the peak concentrations. The final peak of the results in *Figure 1.14* is 3.9 µg/litre, a safe level would be 2.5 and therefore the ratio 2.5/3.9 = 0.64 is applied to the doses, giving 0.48 for the loading dose and 0.19 for the maintenance dose.

In the next run these doses are rounded to 0.5 and 0.2 mg respectively.

```
Run details



Digoxin 0.2mg every 24h for 6 doses oral, loading dose
0.5mg in 3 portions at 8h intervals;

start, primary display, graph;

display and print semilog plot, minC = 0.1, cycles = 2;

stop.
```

The results in *Figure 9.15* show that this regimen is satisfactory, though as the plasma concentrations are still increasing slightly it should be tested by continuation for a further period, to ensure long-term safety.

5.4 Conclusions

As was found with paracetamol, scaling an adult dose for a child by the ratio of body masses, results in underdoses. The ratio of body surface areas gives much better results.

In an elderly man the plasma half-life of digoxin is substantially greater than in a young man. When doses suitable for the young man are given to the 80-year-old, this increase in half-life causes higher plasma concentrations leading to toxic effects.

A suitable regimen for the 80-year-old is obtained by scaling down the doses so that the peaks are below the toxic level.

6. CLINICAL EXAMPLES AND PROBLEMS

In these examples the run details and plots of results are not shown. Sufficient information is given for you to set up the runs and produce your own graphs.

6.1 Gentamicin

6.1.1 *Example*

A 70-kg male, aged 40 years, height 180 cm, with a normal serum creatinine of 0.08 mmol/l (approximately equivalent to a creatinine clearance of 120 ml/min or 7.2 l/h) is receiving 80 mg of gentamicin by i.v. bolus every 8 h. After 48 h, when the steady state can be assumed, he has a pre-dose (trough) plasma concentration of 0.6 mg/l and a post-dose (0.25 h after dose, an approximate peak) concentration of 5.4 mg/l.

Observe the effects of (i) increasing the dose from 80 mg to 120 and to 160 mg; (ii) changing the dosing interval with the 120-mg dose from 8 h to 6 and to 12 h.

Evaluate an effective regimen from these runs.

The five runs can be made successively with bactrack same drug in between. When the dosing interval is changed, the timings of results also have to be changed. The number of doses is set at 7; the run length for the first three runs is 56 h, with *C* results at 0.25 and 8 h after each dose. For the other two runs, lengths and timings of results are adjusted according to the dosing interval. The primary display is a table with a final semilog display.

The results are summarized below. The *C* values in mg/l are for the last dose in each case.

Dose (mg)	Interval (h)	Peak C (mg/l)	Trough C (mg/l)
80	8	5.4	0.6
120	8	8.1	1.0
160	8	10.8	1.3
120	6	8.9	1.8
120	12	7.5	0.3

Peak concentrations are above 8 mg/l for the 160-mg dose and for the 120-mg dose, both 8 and 6 hourly. These doses will provide good anti-bacterial action, without toxicity. In all cases the trough concentrations are below 2 mg/l, again making toxicity unlikely.

If the indication for gentamicin was a life-threatening infection, 6-hourly dosing would be preferable. In the absence of information about the minimum inhibitory concentration for the organism(s) concerned, inadequate concentrations are less likely with the 6-h period.

The regimen of 120 mg every 6 h is therefore chosen.

6.1.2 Problem

A 110-kg, 150-cm, 70-year-old female is thought to have septicaemia caused by gram negative bacteria and she needs to be started on gentamicin given by i.v. bolus. She has a serum creatinine concentration of 0.12 mmol/l, approximately equivalent in this patient to a creatinine clearance of 50 ml/min.

Find (i) the i.v. bolus loading dose necessary to achieve a peak plasma concentration of 8 mg/l; (ii) the time taken after the loading dose is given for the concentration to fall below 3 mg/l; (iii) at the steady state, the dose and dosing interval needed to obtain a peak of 8mg/l and a trough below 3 mg/l.

During her illness, her serum creatinine rises, due to impaired renal function, to a level of 0.2 mmol/l. Perform another run using the dosing schedule already derived to see the effect on the concentration–time profile at the steady state. By increasing the dosing interval in increments of 2 h, find the interval which gives peak concentrations around 8 mg/l and trough concentrations between 1 and 3 mg/l.

6.2 Theophylline

6.2.1 Example

A 38-year-old male presented to an accident and emergency department with acute severe asthma. His weight was 70 kg and height 180 cm. He had been taking inhaled salbutamol and inhaled beclomethasone prior to presentation. In addition to other medication, he was given a loading dose of 6 mg/kg of theophylline, a total dose of theophylline of 400 mg, as a 20-min infusion of aminophylline. (A 250-mg ampoule of aminophylline contains 80%, i.e. 200 mg, of theophylline.)
(i) Observe the effect over 12 h of administering this loading dose without following it with a maintenance infusion. (ii) A maintenance infusion of 0.9 mg/(kg h), approximately equal to 60 mg/h, was started. Observe the effect of this on the plasma concentration–time profile and find the steady-state plasma concentration. (iii) A plasma theophylline concentration measured at 4 h was 14.5 mg/l and increasing. The infusion rate was reduced to 0.6 mg/(kg h) (i.e. 40 mg/h). Re-run the sequence and note the new steady-state concentration.

(i) A single i.v. infusion of 400 mg over 0.33 h and a run of 12 h with results every 1 h shows that the concentration falls below the active level (5 mg/l) at 9 h.
(ii) A run with the above first infusion plus a second infusion of 60 mg/h for 72 h gives $C = 14.5$ at 4 h and a steady-state concentration at 60 h of 21.1 mg/l.

(iii) A run with a maintenance infusion of 40 mg/h for 72 h gives $C = 12.1$ mg/l at 4 h, with a steady-state concentration of 14.1 mg/l at 48 h.

6.2.2 *Problem*

A 50-year-old male, weight 60 kg, height 170 cm, is started on an oral slow-release theophylline preparation containing 180 mg of theophylline, at a dose of one tablet 12 hourly. Assuming that the effective dose is equal to the nominal dose, t_{lag} is 0.7 h, T_1 is 4 h, T_2 is 7 h, G is 0.7 (see Chapter 6, Section 3), how soon will he have reached the steady state and what peak (5 h after dose for this preparation) and trough concentrations will be achieved?

The dose is increased to 300 mg 12-hourly. Find the time to reach the new steady state and the new peak and trough concentrations.

6.3 Lignocaine

6.3.1 *Example*

A 55-year-old man, weight 75 kg, height 170 cm, is admitted to a coronary care unit with a myocardial infarction. He develops frequent runs of ventricular tachycardia and is started on i.v. lignocaine to suppress them. He is given a bolus dose of 100 mg and this is followed immediately by a constant-rate infusion of 2 mg/min (120 mg/h).
(i) Observe the concentration–time profile for the first 6 h, note the duration of sub-therapeutic concentrations; (ii) using an identical maintenance dose, look at the effect on the duration of sub-therapeutic concentrations of a loading dose given as a 200-mg i.v. infusion over 20 min.

In the simulation program, i.v. bolus and infusion doses cannot be given together; however, the bolus can be approximated as a first infusion given over a short period (e.g. 0.02 h).

(i) The dose is 100 mg lignocaine over 0.02 h i.v. infusion with a second infusion of 120 mg/h over 6 h; 6-h run, 24 results at intervals of 0.25 h.
   Sub-therapeutic concentrations (below 2 mg/l) occur up to 0.75 h, the C value increases and at 6 h is 3.3 mg/l, when the steady state is almost attained.
(ii) The sub-therapeutic concentrations are now avoided, the C value rises to 3.4 mg/l at 6 h.

6.3.2 *Problem*

A 70-year-old woman, weight 58 kg, height 160 cm, is receiving an infusion of lignocaine at a rate of 3 mg/min (180 mg/h), following a rapid i.v. infusion loading dose of 100 mg. She becomes nauseated and vomits. Lignocaine toxicity is assumed and her infusion is stopped. The diagnosis is supported by a serum lignocaine concentration well above the toxic level of 6 mg/l.
   Find (i) how long it will take for her plasma concentration to fall below the toxic level; (ii) at what infusion rate the lignocaine should be restarted in order to maintain a therapeutic concentration; (iii) the loading regimen that would achieve a rapid therapeutic concentration of lignocaine.

6.4 **Digoxin**

6.4.1 *Example*

A 58-year-old man, weight 80 kg, height 180 cm, is thought on admission to have been taking digoxin 0.25 mg once daily, but is unable to confirm this because of confusion. He has a supraventricular tachycardia. A digoxin serum concentration was measured to exclude digoxin toxicity and enable further treatment to be planned. The result was 3.8 μg/l, well into the toxic range. Follow the plasma concentration–time profile and note the time from admission to the time when his plasma concentration falls into the non-toxic therapeutic range (1–3 mg/l).

To reach a plasma level of 3.8 μg/l rapidly with this subject in the simulation, 0.5 mg every 8 h is given orally after a loading dose of 1 mg. With this schedule, at 48 h, C is equal to 3.8 μg/l.

To find the time for this concentration to decrease below the 3 μg/l toxic level, the run is continued without doses. After 6 h the concentration reaches 3 μg/l and after 48 h it falls to 1.7 μg/l, still above the minimum active concentration.

6.4.2 *Problem*

A 68-year-old woman, weight 60 kg, height 166 cm, is receiving oral digoxin 0.125 mg once daily (to set up this situation in the simulation she is given an initial loading dose of 0.5 mg in two portions at intervals of 6 h), to control long-standing atrial fibrillation due to rheumatic heart disease. She is admitted to hospital with deteriorating heart failure. Her serum creatinine is found to be rising from its admission level of 0.1 mmol/1 (equivalent in this subject to a *GFR* of 2.7 1/h or 45 ml/min).

Predict the serum creatinine concentration that must be reached before her daily dose of digoxin should be reduced to maintain her in the therapeutic range and to prevent toxic effects. Do this by performing a run over 168 h (1 week) with a serum creatinine concentration of 0.1 mmol/l, increase this value by increments of 0.05 mmol/l, running for a further week with the new value and continuing the process until toxic levels are reached.

The patient's renal function stabilizes at a serum creatinine concentration of 0.25 mmol/l; find the daily dose of digoxin that will maintain her in the therapeutic range.

Drug Kinetic Theory — Mathematical Supplement

In this supplement the theory developed in Chapter 1 and used throughout the book is considered in a more mathematical context. Rate of change and area under the curve are expressed in calculus form; the variation of plasma concentration with time, rate(C) of chapter 1, becomes dC/dt; the area under the C,t curve from zero time to time t_T is represented as the integral:

$$\int_0^{t_T} C \cdot dt$$

1. FIRST-ORDER PROCESSES

1.1 Definitions: the rate equation

A first-order rate process is one in which the rate of change of the concentration of a substance with time is proportional to the concentration. If the process concerned is the elimination of a drug, it may be described by the differential equation

$$dC/dt = -k \cdot C$$

$$(I.1)$$

where dC/dt is the rate of change of C with t, k is the rate constant, taken as positive. The minus sign indicates that C decreases as t increases. The units of k are 1/time; with t in hours, k is in 1/hour, written h^{-1}. From this equation we would like to know the value of C as a direct function of t.

1.2 Solution of the rate equation

Equation (I.1) may be solved by separating the variables (C and t) and integrating:

$$\int dC/C = -k \int dt$$

k may be taken outside the right-hand integral because it is a constant factor. Integration of both sides of the equation then gives $\ln(C)$ for the left side and $-k \cdot t$ for the right, where $\ln(C)$ is the natural logarithm of the concentration. Unless limits are specified for the integrals, an undetermined integration constant, I, has to be included to give the general form:

$$\ln(C) = I - k \cdot t$$

(I.2)

I may be determined by substituting a pair of known values for C and t. For example, for i.v. dose, $C = C_0$ at $t = 0$ and so

$$\ln(C_0) = I$$

and substituting this value of I:

$$\ln(C) = \ln(C_0) - k \cdot t$$

(I.3)

Equation (I.3) is a particular form of the integrated equation (I.2) for the boundary conditions, $C = C_0$ at $t = 0$.

By taking antilogarithms, equation (I.3) becomes

$$C = C_0 \cdot \exp(-k \cdot t)$$

(I.4)

where $\exp()$ denotes the base of natural logarithms, e ($= 2.718$), raised to the power shown in the brackets. C thus declines exponentially from the starting value C_0 towards zero at infinite time.

Converting equation (I.3) to logarithms to the base 10:

$$\log(C) = \log(C_0) - (k/2.3) \cdot t$$

This is the equation of a straight line plot of $\log(C)$ versus t, with slope $-k/2.3$, and intercept on the $\log(C)$ axis of $\log(C_0)$.

1.3 Half-life

The half-life, $t_{1/2}$, of a first-order process is the time taken for C to decrease to half its value. If the starting value is C_0, then from equation (I.3), substituting $C = C_0/2$ at $t = t_{1/2}$:

$$\ln(C_0/2) = \ln(C_0) - k \cdot t_{1/2}$$

therefore:

$$-\ln(2) = -k \cdot t_{1/2}$$

and since $\ln(2) = 0.693$:

$$t_{1/2} = 0.693/k$$

(I.5)

$t_{1/2}$ is therefore independent of concentration and is inversely proportional to the rate constant k.

2. AREA UNDER THE C,t CURVE

The area under the C,t curve is the definite integral:

$$\text{area} = \int_0^{t_1} C \cdot dt$$

(I.6)

where t_1 is the time up to which the area is measured.

2.1 Area and amount of drug

The relationship between area and amount of drug passing through the plasma may be developed as follows.
    If the elimination of drug is first-order with a rate constant k:

$$dC/dt = -k \cdot C$$

If dX_e/dt is the rate of drug elimination in mg/h, dC/dt is the rate of plasma concentration change due to this elimination in mg/(l h) and V is the total volume in which the drug is distributed, then, since amount equals concentration multiplied by volume:

$$dX_e/dt = -V \cdot dC/dt$$

The negative sign appears because X_e, the amount eliminated, is increasing as time increases while C is decreasing.
    Substituting for dC/dt from equation (I.1):

$$dX_e/dt = V \cdot k \cdot C$$

(I.7)

To obtain the total amount of drug $X_{e,1}$ which has passed through the plasma and been eliminated in the period $t = 0$ to $t = t_1$, this equation is integrated between these two times. If k and V are independent of t, they can be taken outside the integral, giving

$$X_{e,1} = k \cdot V \int_0^{t_1} C \cdot dt$$

The integral on the right-hand side is the area, area_1, under the C,t curve up to time t_1 and therefore

$$X_{e,1} = k \cdot V \cdot \text{area}_1$$

(I.8)

2.2 Total area

To assess the total amount of drug which passes through the plasma from a given dose, it is necessary to know the total area under the C,t curve. This area is obtained by integrating C with respect to t between the limits $t = 0$ and $t = \infty$.

$$\text{area}_T = \int_0^{\infty} C \cdot dt$$

From experimental values of C and t, the area, area_N, up to the last result (t_N, C_N) is determined by the trapezium method. The area beyond this point is

$$\text{area}_e = \int_{t_N}^{\infty} C \cdot dt$$

This area may be evaluated by substituting for C from equation (I.4):

$$\text{area}_e = \int_{t_N}^{\infty} C_0 \cdot \exp(-k \cdot t) \cdot dt$$

C_0 is constant and may be taken outside the integral and so, on carrying out the integration, since $\exp(-\infty) = 0$

$$C_0 \int_{t_N}^{\infty} \exp(-k \cdot t) \cdot dt = C_0 [\exp(-k \cdot t)/(-k)]_{t_N}^{\infty} = 0 + C_0 \cdot \exp(-k \cdot t_N)/k$$

From equation (I.4)

$$C_0 \cdot \exp(-k \cdot t_N) = C_N$$

therefore

$$\text{area}_e = C_N/k$$

(I.9)

The total area is

$$\text{area}_T = \int_0^{t_N} C \cdot dt + \int_{t_N}^{\infty} C \cdot dt = \text{area}_N + \text{area}_e$$

$$\text{area}_T = \text{area}_N + C_N/k$$

(I.10)

3. VOLUME OF DISTRIBUTION

The effective volume of distribution following a single dose of a drug varies with time at first and then usually approaches a constant value when the $\log(C), t$ plot becomes linear.

Equation (I.8) gives the time mean value of V:

$$V = X_{e,1}/(k \cdot \text{area}_1)$$

k may be estimated from the slope of the $\log(C), t$ plot in the linear region. If area_1 is the total area under the C, t curve then $X_{e,1}$ is the total amount of drug passing through the plasma. If the route of administration is intravenous, this is the dose D.

$$V = D/(k \cdot \text{area}_T)$$

(I.11)

When the drug is given by the oral or i.m. route, $X_{e,1}$ is the dose multiplied by the bioavailability, F:

$$V = F{\cdot}D/(k{\cdot}\text{area}_T)$$

(I.12)

Equations (I.11) and (I.12) are used to assess the time mean apparent volume of distribution for a drug.

4. CLEARANCE

The clearance of a drug by an elimination route (denoted by subscript 'r') is defined as the rate of elimination by this route in mg/h, $(dX_e/dt)_r$, divided by the plasma concentration, C.

$$Cl_r = (dX_e/dt)_r/C$$

(I.13)

4.1 Renal clearance

If X_u is the amount of drug excreted in the urine up to time t and X is the total amount in the body at this time, then the rate of excretion is dX_u/dt. This rate is equal to minus the rate of reduction of X due to urinary excretion, $-(dX/dt)_u$. The subscript 'u' indicates that this is only part of the change of X with t.

The amount in the body, X, and the plasma concentration, C, taken as representing the overall body fluid concentration of drug, are related by the apparent volume of distribution, V:

$$dX/dt = V{\cdot}dC/dt$$

The rate of urinary excretion is equal to minus the rate of change of X with t due to this excretion:

$$dX_u/dt = -(dX/dt)_u = -V(dC/dt)_u$$

Urinary excretion is usually first-order with respect to plasma concentration and may be expressed in the form

$$(dC/dt)_u = -k_u{\cdot}C$$

and so

$$dX_u/dt = V{\cdot}k_u{\cdot}C$$

(I.14)

where k_u is the urinary excretion rate constant.
The renal clearance Cl_r, is defined by equation (I.13) as the rate of urinary excretion in mg/h, divided by the mean plasma concentration of drug over the period concerned.

$$Cl_r = (dX_u/dt)/C$$

(I.15)

205

Substituting for dX_u/dt from equation (I.14):

$$Cl_r = V \cdot k_u$$

(I.16)

Equation (I.16) means that for situations where V and k_u are constant, the clearance will also be constant, and independent of C and t.

Renal clearance is calculated from experimental results by determining the amount of drug excreted in the urine, ΔX_u mg, over a time interval from say t_1 to t_2 hours. The plasma concentrations C_1 and C_2 at t_1 and t_2, are also determined.

The mean rate of excretion over the interval is then $\Delta X_u/(t_2 - t_1)$ mg/h; the mean plasma concentration is $(C_1 + C_2)/2$ mg/litre. The clearance is therefore

$$Cl_r = [\Delta X_u/(t_2 - t_1)]/[(C_1 + C_2)/2] \text{ l/h}$$

(I.17)

4.2 Total clearance

The total clearance of a drug by all elimination pathways, Cl_T, may be defined using the general definition of clearance (equation I.13) as

$$Cl_T = (dX_e/dt)/C$$

(I.18)

where X_e is the amount eliminated by all mechanisms.

Substituting for dX_e/dt from equation (I.7):

$$Cl_T = V \cdot k$$

(I.19)

This equation is analogous to equation (I.16) for renal clearance. For first-order elimination, since k is constant, Cl_T is also constant.

Total clearance may also be estimated from equation (I.18) expressed as the ratio of the mean rate of elimination over a long period t_T divided by the mean plasma concentration over this period.

Here t_T should be sufficiently long for the drug to be completely eliminated.

The mean rate of elimination is the total amount of drug passing through the plasma (D for the i.v. route or $F \cdot D$ for other routes of administration) divided by t_T. The mean plasma concentration may be expressed by the mean value theorem as

$$C_{mean} = \int_0^{t_T} C \cdot dt/t_T = \text{area}_T/t_T \text{ mg/l}$$

Thus for clearance we have

$$Cl_T = (F \cdot D/t_T)/(\text{area}_T/t_T)$$

t_T cancels, leaving

$$Cl_T = F \cdot D / \text{area}_T$$

(I.20)

For the i.v. route, $F = 1$, and so

$$Cl_T = D / \text{area}_T$$

(I.21)

Hence the total clearance is calculated from experimental results by carrying out a C,t study with dose D, so as to determine the total area under the C,t plot.

4.3 Hepatic clearance

It is not usually possible to determine the hepatic clearance of a drug directly. When the total clearance is due only to urinary excretion and to metabolism in the liver, the hepatic clearance, Cl_h, is estimated as the difference between total and renal clearances.

$$Cl_h = Cl_T - Cl_r$$

(I.22)

5. COMBINED RATE EQUATIONS

5.1 One-compartment model (uncomplicated first-order), i.v. bolus

When the complete volume of distribution is relatively small and the distribution is rapid, the plasma concentration, C, may be taken to be the concentration throughout the distribution volume; no term for the distribution rate is therefore required in the combined rate equation. In this case the drug plasma concentrations are said to follow a one-compartment distribution model, the drug in the plasma and in the outer distribution volume behaves as though it is dissolved in a single fluid compartment. For i.v. bolus dose in its simplest form, the rate equation then contains only two terms: one for metabolism and one for urinary excretion.

$$dC/dt = -k_m \cdot C - k_u \cdot C$$

The 'k' values are first-order rate constants, which may be combined into a single elimination rate constant, k.

$$dC/dt = -(k_m + k_c) \cdot C = -k \cdot C$$

(I.23)

This equation may be integrated as in Section I.2, to give

$$C = C_0 \cdot \exp(-k \cdot t) \text{ where } C = C_0 \text{ at } t = 0$$

(I.24)

In this case, the $\log(C)$,t plot following an i.v. bolus dose is linear.

5.2 Two-compartment model (biphasic), i.v. bolus

Relatively slow attainment of the complete volume of distribution, often found with drugs which are relatively widely distributed, leads to a biphasic, curved $\log(C)$,t plot following i.v. bolus dose (Chapter 1, Section 5.2). The plasma concentrations are then said to follow a two-compartment distribution model, the drug behaving as though it is distributed in two separate fluid compartments.

An additional term has to be put into the combined rate equation to account for the slow transfer between the two volumes V_1 and V_2. The first volume consists of the plasma and tissues and fluids to which the distribution occurs rapidly; the second volume is made up of the tissues and fluids to which distribution occurs more slowly.

The equation is

$$dC/dt = -(k_m + k_u) \cdot C - k_d(C - C_d)$$

C_d is the mean concentration in the second volume and C, the plasma concentration, represents the first volume. k_d is the rate constant for the transfer between the two volumes which continues until $C_d = C$; C_d is less than C during the slow transfer phase.

In the above equation, C_d may be expressed in terms of C and dC/dt by using a conservation equation. With some manipulation, the rate equation may be reduced to an integrable form which gives C in terms of t. The integrated equation has two exponential terms, accounting for the curved $\log(C)$,t plot.

$$C = A \cdot \exp(-\alpha \cdot t) + B \cdot \exp(-\beta \cdot t)$$

(I.25)

α and β are rate constants and α is taken as the larger of the two. The value of α governs the curvature of the early part of a $\log(C)$,t plot (the alpha phase). At longer times $\exp(-\alpha \cdot t)$ becomes negligible and the late time part of the plot (the beta phase) becomes linear with a slope proportional to β.

5.3 Saturable metabolism, i.v. bolus

When a drug has capacity-limited metabolism (Chapter 1, Section 6.1), the Michaelis–Menten equation is used in the combined rate equation, in place of the term for first-order metabolism.

The rate of change of total amount of drug due to saturable metabolism is given by equation (1.3):

$$dX/dt = -V_{max} \cdot C/(K_m + C)$$

The corresponding rate of change of concentration is:

$$(dC/dt)_m = (dX/dt)/V = -(V_{max}/V) \cdot C/(K_m + C)$$

V_{max} is the maximum rate of metabolism in mg/h, V is the apparent volume of distribution and K_m is the Michaelis constant.

To obtain the combined rate equation, a urinary excretion term is added:

$$dC/dt = -(V_m/V)\cdot C/(K_m + C) - k_u\cdot C$$

(I.26)

This equation is not readily integrable to give C as a straightforward function of t. Numerical integration methods are used to solve kinetic equations of this type.

5.4 First-order kinetics, one-compartment distribution, oral route

With drug administration by the oral route, the kinetic effects of slow absorption have to be included in the rate equation.

We designate the total amount of drug absorbed from the oral dose by X_o, which is equal to $F\cdot D$, where F is the bioavailability and D is the dose given.

If X_a is the amount of drug available for absorption and remaining in the dosage form at time t, the rate of absorption of drug from the dosage form is $-dX_a/dt$. If the absorption is a first-order process with a rate constant k_a:

$$dX_a/dt = -k_a\cdot X_a$$

The sign is negative because X_a decreases as t increases.

Separating the variables, integrating and substituting $X_a = X_0$ at $t = 0$ gives

$$X_a = X_0\cdot\exp(-k_a\cdot t)$$

The rate of uptake to the plasma $(dX/dt)_a$ is $-dX_a/dt$:

$$(dX/dt)_a = -dX_a/dt = k_a\cdot X_a$$

The rate of increase of plasma concentration due to this uptake, $(dC/dt)_a$, is $(dX/dt)_a$ divided by the apparent volume of distribution, V:

$$(dC/dt)_a = (dX/dt)_a/V = k_a\cdot X_a/V$$

With first-order elimination, the rate of change of C with t due to elimination is

$$(dC/dt)_e = -k\cdot C$$

Combining absorption and elimination rates:

$$dC/dt = (dC/dt)_a + (dC/dt)_e = k_a\cdot X_a/V - k\cdot C$$

Substituting for X_a:

$$dC/dt = (k_a\cdot X_0/V)\exp(-k_a\cdot t) - k\cdot C$$

(I.27)

This is a first-order linear differential equation in C and t, and may be solved to give C in terms of t. If $C = 0$ at $t = 0$, the result is:

$$C = (X_0/V)[k_a/(k_a - k)][\exp(-k\cdot t) - \exp(-k_a\cdot t)]$$

(I.28)

Equation (I.28) may be used to estimate the mean absorption constant, k_a, from a set of experimental C,t data either by a graphical or by a least-squares method. If the drug exhibits slow distribution, the rate equation (I.27) has to include a distribution function, making the integrated form more complicated.

5.5 Elimination rate constant and half-life, oral route

In equation (I.28), if k_a is greater than k such that at late times $\exp(-k_a \cdot t)$ becomes very small while $\exp(-k \cdot t)$ is still finite, the value of C becomes approximately

$$C = (X_0/V)[k_a/(k_a - k)]\exp(-k \cdot t) = \text{constant} \cdot \exp(-k \cdot t)$$

similar to the equation for i.v. bolus dose. At late times when the absorption is complete, the $\log(C),t$ plot becomes linear and k may be estimated from the slope.

The elimination half-life of the drug is then

$$t_{1/2} = 0.693/k$$

When k and k_a are of similar magnitude, as happens with drugs which are rapidly eliminated, such as ampicillin, the observed late time slope of the $\log(C),t$ plot is influenced by continuing absorption and the plasma half-life estimated from oral dose data is significantly larger than that estimated from i.v. dose data.

6. REPEATED DOSING — THE STEADY STATE

6.1 Mathematical theory

The mathematical theory of the steady state is developed by considering the plasma concentration of a drug at a time t after the Mth repeated dose of D mg; this concentration is made up of the sum of all the concentrations remaining from the doses so far given.

The theory is greatly simplified by assuming that each component of plasma concentration can be expressed in terms of time by a single exponential function. This assumption is approximately true if the dose interval is moderately long and the plasma concentration is assessed towards the end of each interval. Effects due to slow absorption of oral or i.m. doses and due to distribution will then be small and only the exponential term containing the late time elimination constant k will be significant. We may then express C in the form

$$C = A \cdot \exp(-k \cdot t)$$

where A and k are constants. After the first dose, the plasma concentration at time t is thus

$$C_1 = A \cdot \exp(-k \cdot t)$$

If the dosing interval is I_D hours, at time t after the second dose, the concentration remaining from the first dose is $A \cdot \exp[-k(I_D + t)]$; the concentration from the second dose will be $A \cdot \exp(-k \cdot t)$; the total concentration will therefore be

$$C_2 = A \cdot \exp[-k(I_D + t)] + A \cdot \exp(-k \cdot t)$$

The first exponential may be factorized:

$$\exp[-k(I_D + t)] = \exp(-k \cdot I_D) \cdot \exp(-k \cdot t)$$

taking out $A \cdot \exp(-k \cdot t)$ as a factor:

$$C_2 = A \cdot \exp(-k \cdot t)[\exp(-k \cdot I_D) + 1]$$

At time t after the third dose, the concentration remaining from the first dose will be $A \cdot \exp[-k(2 \cdot I_D + t)]$ and by adding this to the amounts remaining from the second and third doses and factorizing as above:

$$C_3 = A \cdot \exp(-k \cdot t)[\exp(-2 \cdot k \cdot I_D) + \exp(-k \cdot I_D) + 1]$$

By analogy, the total plasma concentration after the Mth dose is

$$C_N = A \cdot \exp(-k \cdot t)\{\exp[-(M - 1) \cdot k \cdot I_D] + \exp[-(M - 2) \cdot k \cdot I_D]$$

$$+ \dots + \exp(-2 \cdot k \cdot I_D) + \exp(-k \cdot I_D) + 1\}$$

If the expression in the curly brackets is reversed, it is seen that it is a geometrical progression of M terms with a first term of 1 and a ratio of $\exp(-k \cdot I_D)$, each term being obtained from the previous one by multiplying by this ratio. The sum of such a progression is

$$\text{Sum} = (\text{first term}) \cdot (1 - \text{ratio})/(1 - \text{ratio}^M)$$

In this case

$$\text{Sum} = [1 - \exp(-k \cdot I_D)]/[1 - \exp(-M \cdot k \cdot I_D)]$$

As M is increased, $\exp(-M \cdot k \cdot I_D)$ becomes smaller and ultimately negligible. The value of C in the steady state, at time t after the last dose, is therefore

$$C_{SS} = A \cdot \exp(-k \cdot t)(\text{Sum})$$

$$C_{SS} = A \cdot \exp(-k \cdot t)[1 - \exp(-k \cdot I_D)]$$

$$(I.29)$$

This equation is independent of M, meaning that the next dose, the $(M + 1)$th, will give exactly the same C values at times t after dose as the Mth dose. At this steady state the plasma concentrations in the dosing interval are exactly repeated for each further dose.

6.2 Number of doses and time to steady state

The steady state is reached when $\exp(-M \cdot k \cdot I_D)$ becomes negligible. For practical purposes, in estimating the number of doses to the steady state, N_{SS}, a value of 0.01 is taken as negligible.

The steady-state condition is then

$$\exp(-N_{SS} \cdot k \cdot I_D) < 0.01$$

Taking natural logarithms

$$-N_{SS} \cdot k \cdot I_D < \ln(0.01)$$

and since $\ln(0.01) = -4.61$, this is equivalent to

$$N_{SS} \cdot k \cdot I_D > 4.61$$

$$N_{SS} > 4.61/(k \cdot I_D)$$

Expressing k in terms of plasma half-life, $k = 0.693/t_{1/2}$:

$$N_{SS} > 6.65 \cdot t_{1/2}/I_D$$

(I.30)

For example, with ampicillin, the plasma half-life is 1.5 h, and therefore with repeated doses at 4-h intervals, inequality (I.30) gives

$$N_{SS} > 6.65 \cdot 1.5/4 > 2.5$$

The steady state will therefore be reached after three doses, that is about 8 h after dosing starts.

The time to the steady state, t_{SS}, may be evaluated as follows. The steady state (to within 1%) is reached at the number of doses, N_{SS}, given by inequality (I.30). The first dose is given at zero time and so the N_{SS}th dose is given at time $(N_{SS} - 1) \cdot I_D$, where I_D is the dosing interval.

$$t_{SS} = (N_{SS} - 1) \cdot I_D$$

i.e. using (I.30):

$$t_{SS} = 6.65 \cdot t_{1/2} - I_D$$

(I.31)

For digoxin, the plasma half-life is around 40 h; a dosing interval of 24 h gives

$$N_{SS} > 6.65 \cdot 40/24 > 11.1$$

Twelve doses are thefore required for a close approach to the steady state. Equation (I.31) gives

$$t_{SS} = 6.65 \cdot 40 - 24 = 254 \text{ h}$$

With drugs of long half-life the approach to the steady state is speeded up by giving an initial loading dose (Chapter 9, Section 5.3).

6.3 Prediction of the maintenance dose in a multi-dose regimen

The prediction of the repeated dose D required to give a target mean steady-state concentration C_{SS} has been discussed in Chapter 1, Section 11.

At the steady state, the consequence of the fact that plasma concentrations are exactly repeated over successive dosing intervals is that over the interval, the mean rate of uptake of drug is equal to the mean rate of elimination.

The mean rate of uptake is the amount taken up in the interval divided by the dosing interval:

$$dX_{uptk}/dt = F \cdot D/I_D$$

212

where X_{uptk} is uptake in mg; F is bioavailability; D is dose given at intervals I_D h. The mean rate of elimination is (from equation I.7)

$$dX_e/dt = k \cdot V \cdot C_{SS}$$

where X_e is amount eliminated in mg (X_e increases as t increases and so the sign of the right-hand side of the equation is positive), k is the first-order elimination constant and C_{SS} is the mean steady-state plasma concentration.

Equating the two rates:

$$F \cdot D/I_D = k \cdot V \cdot C_{SS}$$

Rearranging:

$$D = k \cdot V \cdot I_D \cdot C_{SS}/F$$

Substituting for the total clearance from equation (I.19), $Cl_T = k \cdot V$, into the above equation:

$$D = Cl_T \cdot I_D \cdot C_{SS}/F$$

This is equation (1.14) of Chapter 1, Section 11.

Table I.1 Fraction ionized and pH and pK_a

Acids		Bases
	Dissociation equilibria	
$HA = H^+ + A^-$		$B^+ + H_2O = BOH + H^+$
	Dissociation equilibrium constants, K_a	
$K_a = h \cdot i/ui$		$K_a = h \cdot ui/i$
	$pK_a = -\log(K_a)$	
$pK_a = pH - \log(i/ui)$		$pK_a = pH - \log(ui/i)$
	$Z = pH - pK_a$	
$Z = \log(i/ui)$		$Z = \log(ui/i)$
	Take anti-logarithms	
$i/ui = 10^Z$		$ui/i = 10^Z$
	Define fraction ionized, F_{ion}	
$F_{ion} = i/(i + ui)$		$F_{ion} = i/(i + ui)$
	Calculate F_{ion} in terms of Z	
$1/F_{ion} = 1 + ui/i$ $= 1 + 1/10^Z$ $= (10^Z + 1)/10^Z$		$1/F_{ion} = 1 + ui/i$ $= 1 + 10^Z$
$F_{ion} = 10^Z/(10^Z + 1)$		$F_{ion} = 1/(10^Z + 1)$

Equation (1.15) is obtained by using equation (1.12) to replace Cl_T:

$$Cl_T = F \cdot D_1 / area_T(D_1, \text{same route})$$

where the area is total area under a C,t curve following a single dose D_1 given by the same route as the repeated doses.

$$D = D_1 \cdot I_D \cdot C_{SS} / area_T(D_1, \text{same route})$$

Equation (1.15) has the advantage that the value of the bioavailability, F, is not required.

7. IONIZATION OF ACIDS AND BASES

Figure 1.1 (Chapter 1, Section 2.5) shows the fraction ionized F_{ion} for weak acids and bases, plotted against (pH − pK_a). In this section the equations for these plots are developed; since the arguments for acids and bases are similar they are set out side by side in *Table I.1*.

The unionized form of the acid is denoted by HA, which forms an anion A⁻, e.g. acetic acid. The unionized form of the base is denoted by BOH, forming a cation B⁺, e.g. methylamine.

For brevity the molar concentrations [ ], are written h = [H⁺], i = [ionized form], ui = [unionized form]. (pH - pK_a) is denoted by Z.

The plots in Chapter 1, *Figure 1.1* show F_{ion} as a function of Z for the two cases. The patterns of the two functions are illustrated for several values of Z in *Table I.2*.

Table I.2 Some values of F_{ion} for various values of Z

Z	10^Z	pH	F_{ion} (acid)	F_{ion} (base)
-2	0.01	pK_a - 2	0.01	0.99
-1	0.1	pK_a - 1	0.09	0.91
0	1	pK_a	0.50	0.50
1	10	pK_a + 1	0.91	0.09
2	100	pK_a + 2	0.99	0.01

Properties of the Drugs Represented in the Program

Some properties of the drugs on the main drug file of the simulation program are given below. The doses are for adult patients; C_{act}, the estimated minimum active plasma level is in mg/l, as is C_{tox}, the estimated minimum toxic plasma level; $t_{1/2}$ is the beta phase plasma half-life in h, in a normal adult subject; F_b is the fraction of the plasma drug concentration bound to protein, in a normal subject.

1. AMPICILLIN

Ampicillin is an acid of pK_a 2.5, soluble in water and sparingly soluble in chloroform. The acid or its trihydrate is used for oral and i.m. doses, the sodium salt is used for i.v. injection.

As a bactericide, an oral dose is 1000 mg/6 h; toxic effects are diarrhoea, vomiting and convulsions. Hypersensitive subjects show skin rashes and may suffer anaphylactic shock.

$C_{act} = 2$ $\qquad$ $C_{tox} = 30$ $\qquad$ $t_{1/2} = 1.5$ $\qquad$ $F_b = 0.18$

2. ASPIRIN

Aspirin is an acid of pK_a 3.5, sparingly soluble in water and soluble in chloroform; it is rapidly hydrolysed *in vivo* to salicylic acid, pK_a 3.0.

As an analgesic, an oral dose is 300–1000 mg/4 h. For the treatment of rheumatic disease, the oral dose is 900–1200 mg/4 h, to a maximum of 8000 mg daily. Toxic effects include tinnitus and gastro-intestinal bleeding.

The following values apply to total plasma salicylate, i.e. acetylsalicylic acid plus salicylic acid, C_{act} is set for the treatment of rheumatic disease.

$C_{act} = 150$ $\qquad$ $C_{tox} = 300$ $\qquad$ $t_{1/2} = 2.5$ $\qquad$ $F_b = 0.69$

$t_{1/2}$ is for lower doses (up to 400 mg); there is capacity-limited metabolism of salicylic acid and so the half-life increases at higher doses.

3. DIGITOXIN

Digitoxin is a very weak acid of pK_a 10, almost insoluble in water, but soluble in chloroform.

In the treatment of congestive heart failure it is given orally or by the i.v. route. An oral dose is 0.6 mg followed by 0.4 mg/24 h, adjusted individually. Toxic effects include headache, nausea and vomiting.

$$C_{act} = 0.01 \qquad C_{tox} = 0.03 \qquad t_{1/2} = 120 \qquad F_b = 0.95$$

4. INDOMETHACIN

Indomethacin is an acid of pK_a 4.5, practically insoluble in water, but soluble in chloroform.

When used for the relief of pain, an oral dose of 25 mg is given twice daily, increasing as required to a maximum of 200 mg daily. Toxic effects include vomiting, headache and peptic ulceration.

$$C_{act} = 0.5 \qquad C_{tox} = 5 \qquad t_{1/2} = 10 \qquad F_b = 0.95$$

5. KANAMYCIN

Kanamycin is a base of pK_a 7.2, used as the sulphate, a salt which is soluble in water and almost insoluble in chloroform.

As a bactericide, it is administered by the i.m. or i.v. route; it is poorly absorbed from the GIT. Intramuscular and i.v. doses are 700 mg followed by 350–700 mg twice daily, adjusted according to plasma concentrations. Toxic effects include skin rashes and auditory damage which may lead to permanent deafness.

$$C_{act} = 6 \qquad C_{tox} = 30 \qquad t_{1/2} = 2.5 \qquad F_b = 0.01$$

6. NORTRIPTYLINE

Nortriptyline is a base of pK_a 10, used as the hydrochloride, a salt which is soluble in both water and chloroform.

As an anti-depressant, a starting oral dose is 10–25 mg, three times daily; alternatively the summed dose may be given once daily, usually at night. The toxic effects include dry mouth, blurred vision and tachycardia.

$$C_{act} = 0.05 \qquad C_{tox} = 0.25 \qquad t_{1/2} = 24 \qquad F_b = 0.95$$

7. OXPRENOLOL

Oxprenolol is a base of pK_a 9.6 used as the hydrochloride, a salt which is freely soluble in water and slightly soluble in diethylether.

As a beta-blocker in the treatment of hypertension, oxprenolol is administered by the oral route, doses are 120–480 mg daily in two or three divided doses. Toxic effects include vomiting and fatigue.

$$C_{act} = 0.06 \qquad C_{tox} = 3 \qquad t_{1/2} = 1.5 \qquad F_b = 0.8$$

8. PARACETAMOL

Paracetamol is a weak acid of pK_a 9.5, soluble in water and very slightly soluble in chloroform.

In the treatment of pain, oral doses are 500–1000 mg every 4–6 h as required, up to a maximum of 4000 mg daily. Toxic effects are rare with normal doses; overdoses may cause hepatic necrosis.

$$C_{act} = 5 \qquad C_{tox} = 120 \qquad t_{1/2} = 2.5 \qquad F_b = 0$$

The half-life increases in the overdose range due to saturable metabolism and to possible liver damage.

9. PHENOBARBITONE

Phenobarbitone is an acid of pK_a 7.4, slightly soluble in water and soluble in chloroform. It is also used as the sodium salt which is soluble in water and almost insoluble in chloroform.

As an anti-convulsant, it is given by the oral route. Doses are 90–360 mg once daily with higher doses up to a maximum of 600 mg daily if required. Toxic effects include drowsiness, dizziness, headache and ataxia.

$$C_{act} = 10 \qquad C_{tox} = 17 \qquad t_{1/2} = 90 \qquad F_b = 0.5$$

10. PHENYTOIN

Phenytoin is an acid of pK_a 8.3, almost insoluble in water and sparingly soluble in chloroform. The sodium salt, which is soluble in water and almost insoluble in chloroform, is also used.

In the treatment of epilepsy phenytoin is administered by the oral or i.v. route. An oral dose is 300 mg per day, adjusted individually; the saturable metabolism and small therapeutic index cause dosage problems. Toxic effects include ataxia and psychological disturbance.

$$C_{act} = 10 \qquad C_{tox} = 20 \qquad t_{1/2} = 11 \qquad F_b = 0.93$$

The half-life increases markedly with dose in the therapeutic range, due to capacity-limited metabolism.

11. TEMAZEPAM

Temazepam is a very weak base of pK_a 1.6, practically insoluble in water but soluble in chloroform.

For night-time and pre-operative sedation, oral doses are 10–30 mg. A toxic effect is ataxia.

$$C_{act} = 0.3 \qquad C_{tox} = 28 \qquad t_{1/2} = 13 \qquad F_b = 0.97$$

12. GENTAMICIN

Gentamicin is a mixture of similar bases with a mean pK_a of 8.2, used as the mixed sulphate which is freely soluble in water and sparingly soluble in chloroform.

As an antibiotic it is given by the i.m. or i.v. route; it is poorly absorbed from the GIT. Intramuscular and i.v. doses are 120–180 mg initially, followed by 60–160 mg every 8 h, adjusted according to plasma concentrations. Toxic effects include renal damage, vestibular damage and skin rashes.

$C_{act} = 4$ $\qquad$ $C_{tox} = 12$ $\qquad$ $t_{1/2} = 2.5$ $\qquad$ $F_b = 0.25$

13. DIGOXIN

Digoxin is a very weak acid of pK_a 10 and is almost insoluble in water; it is slightly soluble in chloroform.

In the treatment of atrial fibrillation it is given by the oral or i.v. route; oral divided doses of 0.75–1 mg are given initially, followed by 0.0625–0.5 mg daily, adjusted individually. Toxic effects are similar to those of digitoxin (Section 3).

$C_{act} = 0.001$ $\qquad$ $C_{tox} = 0.003$ $\qquad$ $t_{1/2} = 40$ $\qquad$ $F_b = 0.3$

14. THEOPHYLLINE

Theophylline is weakly amphoteric, as an acid the pK_a is 8.6, as a base the pK_a is less than 1. It is sparingly soluble in water and chloroform. The presence of the organic base ethylenediamine makes it freely soluble in water and it is often formulated as mixture of theophylline and ethylenediamine, called aminophylline. Aminophylline contains about 80% of theophylline.

For rapid effect in the treatment of bronchial asthma, 250–500 mg of aminophylline is injected i.v. over 15 min; oral doses are 180–600 mg of theophylline as a slow-release formulation, twice daily. Toxic effects include dyspepsia, nausea and vomiting and, rarely, serious cardiac arrhythmias and convulsions.

$C_{act} = 5$ $\qquad$ $C_{tox} = 30$ $\qquad$ $t_{1/2} = 9$ $\qquad$ $F_b = 0.4$

15. LIGNOCAINE

Lignocaine is a base of pK_a 7.9, used as the hydrochloride, a salt which is very soluble in water and soluble in chloroform.

As an anti-arrhythmic drug it is given by the i.v. route, with an initial injection (100 mg or more) followed by 3 mg/min infusion, adjusted individually. There is a large first-pass effect when it is given orally, resulting in the formation of a toxic metabolite, and therefore the oral route is not used. Toxic effects include nausea, vomiting and convulsions.

$C_{act} = 2$ $\qquad$ $C_{tox} = 6$ $\qquad$ $t_{1/2} = 1.5$ $\qquad$ $F_b = 0.7$

16. CARBAMAZEPINE

Carbamazepine is a base of pK_a 9, practically insoluble in water but soluble in chloroform.

As an anti-convulsant, oral doses are 100–400 mg twice daily at first, increasing as required. Toxic effects include nausea, headache, drowsiness, double vision, dizziness and ataxia.

$C_{act} = 4$ $\qquad$ $C_{tox} = 10$ $\qquad$ $t_{1/2} = 35$ $\qquad$ $F_b = 0.73$

17. BENZYLPENICILLIN

Benzylpenicillin is an acid of pK_a 2.7, used as a salt, which is very soluble in water but practically insoluble in chloroform.

As an antibiotic it is administered by the i.m. or i.v. route; when given orally only about 30% of the dose is absorbed, the remainder being inactivated by gastric acid. Intramuscular doses are given at 6-h intervals to a daily total of 300–6000 mg. In life-threatening infections, it is given by i.v. bolus dose of 1200 mg every 2 h. Toxic effects include anaphylactic shock, convulsions, rashes and bone marrow depression.

$C_{act} = 2$ $\qquad$ $C_{tox} = 100$ $\qquad$ $t_{1/2} = 1$ $\qquad$ $F_b = 0.55$

18. THIOPENTONE

Thiopentone is an acid of pK_a 7.6, freely soluble in chloroform, it is used as the sodium salt, which is freely soluble in water and almost insoluble in diethylether.

As a short-acting anaesthetic, it is given as an i.v. bolus of 250 mg, the onset of anaesthesia is within a few seconds and the duration is about 5 min. Toxic effects include respiratory depression and hypotension.

$C_{act} = 25$ $\qquad$ $C_{tox} = 80$ $\qquad$ $t_{1/2} = 8$ $\qquad$ $F_b = 0.8$

19. ATENOLOL

Atenolol is a base of pK_a 9.6.

As a beta-blocker in the treatment of hypertension, 50–100 mg of atenolol is given daily as a single dose by the oral route. Toxic effects include cold extremities and fatigue.

$C_{act} = 0.15$ $\qquad$ $C_{tox} = 5$ $\qquad$ $t_{1/2} = 8$ $\qquad$ $F_b = 0.05$

20. DIAMORPHINE

Diamorphine, used as the hydrochloride, is a base of pK_a 7.6, which is rapidly hydrolysed *in vivo* to acetylmorphine and then to morphine. The longer-term effects are due to morphine. The hydrochloride is soluble in both water and chloroform.

As a narcotic analgesic it is used when the i.m., i.v. or subcutaneous routes are required. An i.m. dose is 10 mg every 4 h. Toxic effects include nausea and vomiting. The data below are for total morphine following dosing with diamorphine.

$C_{act} = 0.01$ $\qquad$ $C_{tox} = 0.2$ $\qquad$ $t_{1/2} = 2$ $\qquad$ $F_b = 0.35$

APPENDIX III

The Subject Factors

1. THE SUBJECT FACTOR LIST

The nine subject factors used in the MuPharm simulation are:

1. plasma volume, l
2. rate constant for transfer, liver to main plasma, h^{-1}
3. effective gastric pH
4. volume of distribution, l
5. hepatic function, relative to standard
6. interactive hepatic function
7. urine flow rate, l/h
8. urine pH
9. glomerular filtration rate, l/h

These factors are referred to subsequently as sf(n), where n is the factor number in the above list.

All the subject factors except sf(5) may be changed interactively through the CHANGE sub-menu (Chapter 4, Section 3.4).

sf(5) is a hepatic function which has the value 1.0 for the standard subject and which is set automatically in the program for other subjects. sf(6) is a hepatic function with a value of 1.0 for all subjects which may be set by the user so as to simulate a loss of hepatic function.

2. VALUES OF THE FACTORS FOR THE STANDARD SUBJECT

The standard subject is a 25-year-old male, body mass 70 kg, height 183 cm.

2.1 sf(1)

According to Wasserman et al. [*J. Lab. Clin. Med.* (1951) **37**, 342], the plasma volume per kg body mass, determined by the dyestuff dilution method for a wide range of male and female adults treated as one group, ranges from 0.031 to 0.054 l/kg with a mean of 0.042.

For 70-kg subjects, the range is therefore 2.2–3.8 l with a mean of 2.94. In addition to its dependence on total body mass, plasma volume is also a function of height and of the proportion of fat in the body mass. Since our standard subject is an active, tall, lean young man, his plasma volume should be near the top of the range and a value of 3.6 l has been taken for sf(1).

When a short, portly, 70-kg middle-aged subject is set up in the simulation, sf(1) is adjusted automatically in the program to a value near the bottom of the range for 70-kg subjects.

2.2 sf(2)

This rate constant for transfer of drug from the liver to the main plasma volume is only used for oral doses. It represents the liver blood flow and governs the extent of the first-pass effect. It has been calibrated for the standard subject using the first-pass effect with oral nortriptyline; a value of 16 h^{-1} has been adopted.

Changes to sf(2) may be used to simulate the effect of reduced cardiac output on the first-pass metabolism of a drug. Reduction below 5 h^{-1} may cause instability in the calculations.

2.3 sf(3)

The effective gastric pH is the pH of the absorbing surface rather than the pH of the gastric contents; a value of 3.5 is used.

2.4 sf(4)

This factor is the physical volume of distribution outside the plasma. A value of 37 l has been taken for this volume for the standard subject.

In the case of overweight subjects receiving drugs with small lipid solubility, sf(4) is modified so as to limit the distribution of the drug.

In all cases, sf(4) is multiplied by a drug factor, the distribution ratio, df(9), to determine the apparent volume of distribution outside the plasma. When the drug has limited distribution, this ratio is less than 1. When the drug is more widely distributed to the intracellular volume and to lipid, this ratio will be greater. When the drug is strongly bound outside the plasma, the ratio may be much greater than 1, giving an apparent volume of distribution substantially larger than the physical volume. For example, nortriptyline in a 70-kg subject has an apparent volume of distribution of over 1000 l.

2.5 sf(5)

The hepatic function relative to the standard subject is adjusted automatically in the simulation program for individual specified subjects. It cannot be altered in the dialogue.

2.6 sf(6)

The interactive hepatic function is normally 1.0 for all subjects; it may be altered so as to simulate liver dysfunction, e.g. a 40% reduction of function for any subject would result from setting sf(6) to 0.6.

2.7 sf(7)

The urine flow rate is taken as 0.066 l/h. Diuresis may be simulated by increasing this factor.

2.8 sf(8)

The urine pH is set at 5.5. The effect of treatment with ammonium chloride so as to acidify the urine may be simulated by reducing this value; the effect of treatment with sodium bicarbonate so as to render the urine alkaline is simulated by increasing sf(8).

2.9 sf(9)

The glomerular filtration rate is taken as 7.5 l/h. Kidney dysfunction may be simulated by reducing this rate, e.g. a 40% reduction in renal function for the standard subject would be set up by reducing sf(9) from 7.5 to $0.6 \times 7.5 = 4.5$ l/h.

3. VALUES OF THE FACTORS FOR OTHER SUBJECTS

When the user sets up a new subject in the dialogue, age, mass, height and sex are specified in reply to dialogue requests. sf(1), sf(4), sf(5), sf(7) and sf(9) are all recalculated in the program to comply with the subject characteristics set by the user. Values of these five subject factors are assessed automatically for various age and sex groups.

The user may of course make further changes in the factors through the CHANGE sub-menu, so as to simulate particular patients.

The characteristics and factors for preset subjects may be stored in additional subject files, as described in Appendix VII.

The Drug Factors

There are 18 drug factors, with one, df(6), spare. All except df(1) and df(2) can be altered by the user through the CHANGE menu.

1. THE DRUG FACTOR LIST

1. pK_a
2. acid-base index, 1 for acid, 2 for base
3. rate constant for absorption from the GIT, h^{-1}
4. rate constant for absorption from an i.m. deposit, h^{-1}
5. fraction of the dose which is absorbed from the GIT
6. spare, set at zero
7. fraction bound to plasma protein
8. rate constant for distribution, h^{-1}
9. distribution ratio
10. rate constant for first-order metabolism, h^{-1}
11. maximum rate for capacity-limited metabolism, mg/h
12. Michaelis constant, capacity-limited metabolism, mg/l
13. rate constant for enzyme induction, kilohour^{-1}
14. renal tubular function
15. fraction taken up in the plasma from an i.m. deposit
16. minimum plasma concentration for toxic effects, mg/l
17. lethal plasma concentration, mg/l
18. minimum plasma concentration for drug activity, mg/l
19. concentration units, 1 for mg/l, 2 for µg/l

2. FURTHER DESCRIPTIONS OF SOME FACTORS

Most of the factors, referred to in the text as df(n), are self-explanatory; their places in the structure of the simulation model are outlined in Appendix V. Further details for some of the factors are given below.

2.1 df(13)

Enzyme induction occurs with some drugs over a long period. As a result, the mean steady-state plasma concentration in a multidosing schedule decreases with time. This is a slow effect and so df(13) is given in kilohour^{-1}. A value of 1.0 for df(13) means a half-time for the increase of the metabolic rate constant of 693 h or 29 days.

2.2 df(14)

The renal tubular function is a dividing factor in the calculation of the rate of urinary excretion of the drug (it is the *RTF* of Chapter 1, Section 7.2). A large value means that the drug is only slowly excreted in the urine, due to renal tubular reabsorption. A small value of 1.0 or less means that the drug is rapidly excreted in the urine, often due, as with the penicillins, to renal tubular secretion.

2.3 df(19)

This factor determines the plasma concentration units for output in the table of results and in the graphs. It has been found that the two sets of units, mg/l and μg/l, adequately cover all the drugs on the list.

2.4 Lag times

In addition to the 19 drug factors, lag times for the oral and i.m. routes are set for each drug. They are given values for usual preparations of the drug, or zero.

3. NUMERICAL VALUES FOR THE DRUGS ON THE MAIN LIST

The drug factors and lag times for the 20 drugs which are available from the main list are given below, in the form in which files for new drugs set up by the user should be arranged (Appendix VI).

The first line gives the drug name; the second consists of df(1) to df(10), the numbers are in 'free format', which means that they are set out with the required precision, and are separated by spaces; as they are read in as real numbers they all have to be given decimal points, including the zeros. The third line consists of df(11)–df(19) and the two lag times — oral and i.m.

```
ampicillin

2.5 1. .6 1.4 .5 0. .18 1.6 .22 .65

0. 0. 0. .65 .75 30. 700. 2. 1. .2 .2

aspirin

3.5 1. 3. 0. .9 0. .69 3. .3 0.

150. 23. 0. 20.8 0. 300. 1500. 150. 1. .2 0.

digitoxin

10. 1. 2. 0. .7 0. .95 20. .8 .04

0. 0. 0. 9. 0. .03 .3 .01 2. 0.5 0.
```

indomethacin

4.5 1. 0.6 0. 1. 0. .95 .5 .5 1.25

0. 0. 0. .8 0. 5. 50. .5 2. 0. 0.

kanamycin

7.2 2. 0. 1.5 0. 0. .01 20. .4 0.

0. 0. 0. 1.3 1. 30. 440. 6. 1. 0. .15

nortriptyline

10. 2. .05 0. 1. 0. .945 12. 20. 8.

0. 0. 0. .4 0. .25 2. .05 2. 0. 0.

oxprenolol

9.6 2. .8 0. 1. 0. .8 18. 1.1 6.5

0. 0. 0. 2.78 0. 3. 15. .06 2. .15 0.

paracetamol

9.5 1. 1. 0. 1. 0. 0. 10. 1.3 0.

600. 30. 0. 22.2 0. 120. 500. 5. 1. 0. 0.

phenobarbitone

7.4 1. 0.5 .4 1. 0. .5 3.5 .8 .026

0. 0. 1. 25. .95 17. 47. 10. 1. .15 0.

phenytoin

8.3 1. .7 .14 1. 0. .93 50. 1. 0.

18. 7. 0. 8.3 .5 20. 70. 10. 1. 0. 0.

temazepam

1.6 2. .2 0. 0.9 0. .974 1.0 0.9 1.2

0. 0. 0. 2.2 0. 28. 140. .3 2. 0. 0.

gentamicin

8.2 2. 0. 7.0 0. 0. 0.25 25.0 0.3 0.

0. 0. 0. 1.3 0.98 12. 440. 4. 1. 0. 0.15

digoxin

10. 1. .2 0. 0.9 0. 0.3 5.5 9. .3

0. 0. 0. 0.8 0. .003 .15 .001 2. 0. 0.

theophylline

8.6 1. 1. 0. 1. 0. .4 5. .75 .65

0. 0. 0. 9.3 0. 30. 100. 5.0 1. 0. 0.

lignocaine

7.9 2. 0. .5 0. 0. .7 40. 2. 12.

0. 0. 0. 1.7 .9 6. 14. 2. 1. 0. 0.

carbamazepine

9. 2. .05 0. 1. 0. .73 1. 1.7 .44

0. 0. 1.5 18. 0. 10. 40. 4. 1. 0. 0.

benzylpenicillin

2.7 1. 0. 1.6 0. 0. .55 3. .18 0.8

0. 0. 0. .26 .8 100. 700. 2.0 1. 0. 0.

thiopentone

7.6 1. .3 0. .8 0. .8 10.5 2.5 0.

250. 24. 0. 55.6 0. 80. 200. 25. 1. 0. 0.

atenolol

9.6 2. .31 0. .55 0. .05 9. 1.6 .03

0. 0. 0. 1.2 0. 5. 15. .15 2. .9 0.

diamorphine

8. 2. 0. .47 0. 0. .35 21. 3.3 18.

0. 0. 0. .7 1. .2 .75 .01 2. 0. 0.15

The Design and Implementation of the Mathematical Model of Human Drug Kinetics

1. THE RATE EQUATION

The general rate equation describes the rate of change with time of the amount X mg of drug in the plasma, in terms of a set of subject factors $sf(n)$, and drug factors $df(n)$, the dose D and the route of administration. In functional terms, we might denote this complex relationship in the general form

$$dX/dt = f\{sf(n), df(n), D, \text{route}\}$$

This equation is integrated numerically using increments in t of 0.01 h, small enough to allow simple integration using Euler's method and avoiding the need for more complex integration formulae such as those of Runge-Kutta. The time increment is held constant throughout a run and is called the iteration interval t_I. Its value may be altered interactively at the start of a run.

The increment in X at each iteration is

$$\Delta X = f\{sf(n), df(n), D, \text{route}\} \cdot t_I$$

$$(V.1)$$

Figure V.1 is a diagram showing the processes involved in the simulation model for the i.v. and i.m. routes.

2. INTRAVENOUS BOLUS DOSE

2.1 Input

With rapid i.v. administration, the whole dose D goes directly into the plasma at the start of the run. The input function *UPTK* is therefore

$$UPTK = D \text{ at } t = 0 \quad UPTK = 0 \text{ at } t > 0$$

$$(V.2)$$

In the subsequent iterations, distribution, metabolism and urinary excretion occur and the amounts of drug handled by these processes at each iteration are calculated. They are denoted by ΔX_d, ΔX_m and ΔX_u respectively.

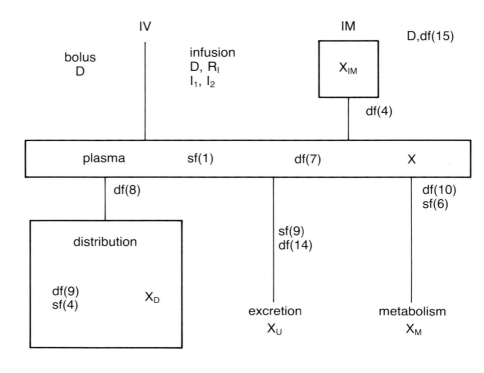

Figure V.1 Intravenous and intramuscular dose, first-order metabolism.

2.2 Distribution

The distribution of drug from the plasma is treated as a first-order, reversible exchange of drug between the plasma and the effective volume of distribution outside the plasma. The rate of the forward process from drug in the plasma to the outer volume is

$$(dX_d/dt)_F = df(8) \cdot X$$

where df(8) is the first-order rate constant for distribution.

The rate of the reverse process is

$$(dX_d/dt)_B = df(8) \cdot sf(1) \cdot X_d / \{sf(4) \cdot df(9)\}$$

sf(1) is the plasma volume of the subject; X_d is the amount of drug currently in the outer volume; sf(4) is the physical volume of distribution outside the plasma for the subject; df(9) is the partition ratio for drug distribution between plasma and outer volume.

sf(4) is modified in overweight subjects for drugs of small lipid solubility, so as to limit the effective volume of distribution.

The net rate of distribution from the plasma is

$$dX_d/dt = (dX_d/dt)_F - (dX_d/dt)_B$$

so that the increment in X_d during each iteration is

$$\Delta X_d = df(8) \cdot \{X - sf(1) \cdot X_d/[sf(4) \cdot df(9)]\} \cdot t_I$$

$$(V.3)$$

ΔX_d is worked out for each iteration, starting with $X_d = 0$ at $t = 0$; the total value of X_d at any time is calculated by adding together the increments ΔX_d up to that time.

2.3 Metabolism

Metabolism is treated as a first-order process for most of the drugs:

$$\Delta X_m = df(10) \cdot sf(6) \cdot X \cdot t_I$$

$$(V.4)$$

where df(10) is the first-order rate constant for drug metabolism and sf(6) is the hepatic function set by the user to simulate a loss of function; sf(6) has a normal value of 1.0 for all subjects (Appendix III).

Some drugs, e.g. aspirin and phenytoin, exhibit capacity-limited, saturable metabolism. The metabolism is then described by a form of the Michaelis–Menten equation, giving the following expression for ΔX_m:

$$\Delta X_m = df(11) \cdot sf(5) \cdot sf(6) \cdot X \cdot t_I/\{df(12) \cdot sf(1) + X\}$$

$$(V.5)$$

where df(11) is the maximum rate of metabolism in mg/h; df(12) is the plasma concentration at which the rate is half the maximum (K_m); sf(1) is the plasma volume for the subject; sf(5) is the hepatic function for the subject set automatically in the program (Appendix III).

In the simulation, the metabolism is treated as either first-order or saturable; if df(10) is non-zero then df(11) and df(12) are set to zero; if df(11) and df(12) are non-zero then df(10) is set to zero.

2.4 Urinary excretion

Urinary excretion of unchanged drug is treated as a first-order process acting on the concentration of unbound drug in the plasma. The rate constant is governed by the glomerular filtration rate for the subject, sf(9) l/h, modified by the renal tubular function for the drug, df(14) (see Chapter 1, Section 7.2). The total plasma concentration is equal to the plasma amount, X, divided by the plasma volume, sf(1).

The concentration of unbound drug is then $\{X/\mathrm{sf}(1)\}\cdot\{1-\mathrm{df}(7)\}$ and

$$\Delta X_u = \{\mathrm{sf}(9)/\mathrm{df}(14)\}\cdot\{1-\mathrm{df}(7)\}\cdot\{X/\mathrm{sf}(1)\}\cdot t_I$$

(V.6)

df(14) is a measure of the net effect of absorption and secretion in the kidney tubules. If there is a net absorption, df(14) has a relatively high value, which acts to decrease the value of ΔX_u; if there is net secretion, df(14) has a low value.

2.5 Total amounts of drug after each iteration

The increments in X_d, X_m and X_u are calculated at each iteration using equations (V.3), (V.4) or (V.5), and (V.6).

At $t = 0$ the starting values for i.v. bolus dose are:

$$X = \mathrm{D}; \quad X_d = 0; \quad X_m = 0; \quad X_u = 0$$

At the end of each iteration, the total amounts are updated by the increments, giving:

$$X_d = X_d{}' + \Delta X_d$$

$$X_m = X_m{}' + \Delta X_m$$

$$X_u = X_u{}' + \Delta X_u$$

(V.7)

The primed symbols on the right-hand side of these equations indicate the values at the start of the iteration.

The overall change in X, the amount of drug in the plasma, is recalculated at each iteration from the other three increments:

$$\Delta X = -\Delta X_d - \Delta X_m - \Delta X_u$$

(V.8)

and the new value of X is then calculated as

$$X = X' + \Delta X$$

(V.9)

At the end of each time interval set by the user for output of results, the plasma concentration is calculated:

$$C = X/\mathrm{sf}(1)$$

(V.10)

As the run proceeds, this concentration may be displayed in a table, together with the current values of t, X_d, X_m, X_u and an estimate of the response of the subject to the drug, or as a graph or in the form of a disposition diagram.

3. INTRAVENOUS INFUSION

The treatment of i.v. infusion differs only from the bolus dose in having a different input function.

With a single i.v. infusion, the user sets a total dose, D, and the duration of the infusion, I_1. This duration is equivalent to $N_1 = I_1/t_I$ iteration intervals. For a constant rate infusion the uptake function is the dose per interval:

$$UPTK = D/N_1 \text{ for } N < = N_1; \quad UPTK = 0 \quad \text{for } N > N_1$$

$$(V.11)$$

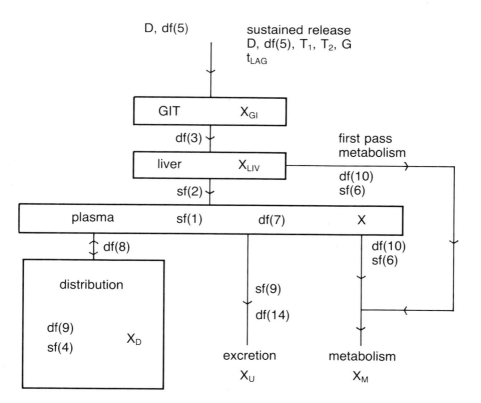

Figure V.2 Oral dose, first-order metabolism.

Equation (V.8) for the increment in X has to take into account the input of drug at each iteration interval. It is modified to

$$\Delta X = UPTK - \Delta X_d - \Delta X_m - \Delta X_u$$

(V.12)

and equation (V.9) is used for the total amount of drug in the plasma.

As the model is set up, when a second infusion is given it follows the first infusion; the user specifies an infusion rate, R_I mg/h, and a duration, I_2, following the end of the first infusion.

The dose per iteration in this second period is $R_I \cdot t_I$ and is continued for $N_2 = I_2/t_I$ iterations. The input function for both infusions is therefore

$$UPTK = D/N_1 \quad \text{for } N <= N_1$$

$$UPTK = R_I \cdot t_I \quad \text{for } N_1 < N <= (N_1 + N_2)$$

$$UPTK = 0 \quad \text{for } N > (N_1 + N_2)$$

where:

$$N_1 = I_1/t_I \text{ and } N_2 = I_2/t_I$$

4. ORAL DOSE

Figure V.2 is a diagram showing the simulation processes for the oral route.

4.1 First-pass effect

The input of drug from the plasma following an oral dose is complicated by the first-pass effect, which results from the direct transfer of absorbed drug from the gastro-intestinal tract (GIT) to the liver via the portal circulation. The newly absorbed drug is therefore partly metabolized before it is distributed outside the plasma.

This effect is taken into account in the simulation model by introducing two further amounts of drug when an oral dose is prescribed. These amounts are X_{GI}, the amount remaining in the GIT, and X_{liv}, the amount in the liver.

The amount of drug available for absorption from an oral dose of D mg is $D \cdot \text{df}(5)$, where df(5) is the fraction absorbed. This amount is considered to go straight into the GIT, from which it is transferred to the liver by a first-order process. In the liver, partial metabolism occurs and the remainder of the drug goes to the main plasma volume, where it undergoes distribution, metabolism and excretion as with i.v. doses.

df(3) is the absorption rate constant and ΔX_{GI} per iteration is estimated as

$$\Delta X_{GI} = -\text{df}(3) \cdot X_{GI} \cdot t_I$$

(V.13)

The starting value for X_{GI} at $t = 0$ is $X_{GI} = D \cdot df(5)$.

The rate of entry of newly absorbed drug to the liver is expressed as

$$dX_{liv}/dt = df(3) \cdot X_{GI} = -dX_{GI}/dt$$

The rate of formation of metabolite from newly absorbed drug in the liver, assuming first-order metabolism, is denoted by

$$(dX_m/dt)_1 = df(10) \cdot X_{liv}$$

$df(10)$ is the metabolic rate constant.

The rate of input of intact, newly absorbed drug to the plasma is

$$dX/dt = sf(2) \cdot X_{liv}$$

$sf(2)$ is the rate constant for transfer of the drug from the liver to the general circulation. This rate constant is related to the liver blood flow and hence to the cardiac output of the subject.

From these considerations, an expression to calculate ΔX_{liv} at each iteration may be developed. However, when this is done and X_{liv} is assessed in the numerical integration, there is a failure to conserve the drug due to the rapid processes in the liver.

In order to avoid this effect, X_{liv} is estimated after each iteration using the conservation equation

$$X_{liv} = D \cdot df(5) - X_{GI} - X - X_d - X_m - X_u$$

$$(V.14)$$

The starting values at $t = 0$ are

$$X_{GI} = D \cdot df(5) \quad X_{liv} = X = X_d = X_m = X_u = 0$$

The change in plasma amount (ΔX_a) due to entry of newly absorbed drug is the input function *UPTK*:

$$UPTK = (\Delta X_a) = sf(2) \cdot X_{liv} \cdot t_I$$

$$(V.15)$$

4.2 Metabolism

The amount of drug metabolized per iteration due to the first-pass effect is:

$$\Delta X_{m,1} = df(10) \cdot sp(5) \cdot X_{liv} \cdot t_I$$

In addition, there is an amount metabolized due to the drug in the general circulation:

$$\Delta X_{m,2} = df(10) \cdot sp(5) \cdot X \cdot t_I$$

so that the total amount metabolized at each iteration is the sum of these two contributions:

$$\Delta X_m = df(10)\cdot sp(5)\cdot (X + X_{liv})\cdot t_I$$

(V.16)

When metabolism is by a limited-capacity rate process, an approximate expression for ΔX_m is used:

$$\Delta X_m = df(11)\cdot sp(5)\cdot (X + X_{liv})\cdot t_I/\{df(12)\cdot sf(1) + X + X_{liv}\}$$

(V.17)

4.3 Distribution and excretion, total change in X

The expressions for ΔX_d and ΔX_u are the same as equations (V.3) and (V.6). The total change in plasma amount per iteration is therefore made up of the input function, equation (V.15), and the disposition functions, equation (V.8).

$$\Delta X = sf(2)\cdot X_{liv}\cdot t_I - \Delta X_d - \Delta X_m - \Delta X_u$$

(V.18)

4.4 Lag time

The time after an oral dose before a detectable amount of drug appears in the plasma, t_{lag}, is taken into account in the model by shifting the time origin from $t = 0$ to $t = t_{lag}$. This shift is not done in the course of the numerical integration, but is applied to the times for which the user has requested a print-out of results.

5. ORAL SUSTAINED-RELEASE PREPARATIONS

The treatment of oral sustained release is similar to that for i.v. infusion except that the rate controlling drug input is now that from the preparation to the GIT.

The user supplies the total dose, D, the durations of two consecutive release periods, T_1 and T_2, and the fraction G of the available dose which is released in the first release period.

At $t = 0$, X_{GI} and all the other X values are set to zero. The number of intervals of iteration in the first release period is $N_1 = T_1/t_I$ and the amount of drug released in each iteration interval in this first period is $G\cdot D\cdot f(5)/N_1$. In the second release period, the number of iterations is $N_2 = T_2/t_I$, and the amount of drug released per iteration is $(1-G)\cdot D\cdot f(5)/N_2$.

The uptake, $UPTK_{GI}$, of drug which is input to the GIT per iteration as a function of iteration number N is therefore

$$UPTK_{GI} = G\cdot D\cdot f(5)/N_1 \text{ for } N <= N_1$$

$$UPTK_{GI} = (1 - G)\cdot D\cdot f(5)/N_2 \text{ for } N_1 < N <= (N_1 + N_2)$$

(V.18)

$$UPTK_{GI} = 0 \text{ for } N > (N_1 + N_2)$$

The positive increments $UPTK_{GI}$ are applied to X_{GI} at each iteration, giving the equation

$$\Delta X_{GI} = UPTK_{GI} - \text{df}(3) \cdot X_{GI} \cdot t_I$$

where the negative term is from equation (V.13), expressing the loss from the GIT due to absorption.

The other X values, apart from X_{liv}, are calculated by the equations in Section 4.

Equation (V.14) for X_{liv} is modified so that the first term on the right-hand side is the total amount of drug which has thus far been released from the preparation. A tally of this amount, X_{rel}, is updated at each iteration.

$$X_{liv} = X_{rel} - X_{GI} - X - X_d - X_m - X_u$$

(V.19)

The lag time effect is taken into account in the same way as in Section 4.4.

6. INTRAMUSCULAR ROUTE

After i.m. administration, the drug is absorbed directly into the plasma and no first-pass effect occurs. It is not therefore necessary to have a separate liver unit as was required for the oral route.

Absorption from the i.m. deposit is taken to be a first-order process. The possibilities of incomplete absorption and of lag time are taken into account.

The input function to the plasma, per iteration, is

$$UPTK = \text{df}(4) \cdot X_{i.m.} \cdot t_I$$

$X_{i.m.}$ is the current amount of drug available for absorption. The starting value for $X_{i.m.}$ at $t = 0$ is $D \cdot \text{df}(15)$, where $\text{df}(15)$ is the fraction taken up into the plasma from the i.m. dose D. The change of amount of drug available for absorption per iteration, $\Delta X_{i.m.}$, is estimated from

$$\Delta X_{i.m.} = -UPTK$$

$\text{df}(4)$ is the first-order rate constant for absorption from the i.m. deposit.

For description of the disposition of the drug, ΔX_d is calculated with equation (V.3); ΔX_m is assessed with equation (V.4) or (V.5); ΔX_u is found with equation (V.6); the total amounts X_d, X_m, and X_u are assessed with equations (V.7); ΔX, the increment per iteration in the plasma amount, is found from equation (V.12), and the total amounts at each iteration are calculated by summing increments, as in equations (V.7) and (V.9), with starting values, $X = X_d = X_m = X_u = 0$.

The lag time for the i.m. dose is treated in the same way as for the oral dose (Section 4.4).

7. REPEATED DOSES

When doses are repeated, the drug input functions are reintroduced into the calculations, starting at iterations corresponding to the times for the administration of new doses set by the user. The values of X, X_d, X_m and X_u are carried forward from the end of the calculations made in the previous dosing interval.

8. OTHER SUBJECT AND DRUG FACTORS

8.1 pK_a, acid–base index, gastric pH

df(1) is the pK_a of a drug; df(2) is the acid–base index, 1 for acid and 2 for base; sf(3) is the effective stomach pH for absorption.

These three factors are used in a section of the simulation model which assesses the effect of change in stomach pH on absorption rate.

In this section the change of pH governs changes in the absorption constant from the GIT, df(3), and in the fraction of the dose absorbed, df(5). The changes are restricted to between 75% and 133% of the normal values, bearing in mind that these drug factors cover the whole absorption from the GIT.

The expressions used are based on the fractions of drug ionized at different pH values. The calculations are summarized below; al stands for antilogarithm, with subscripts 'O' and 'N' to indicate old and new values, before and after the change in pH respectively.

For an anionic (acidic) drug, df(2) = 1:

$$al_O = 10^{(pH_O - pK)} \qquad al_N = 10^{(pH_N - pK)}$$

(V.20)

For a cationic (basic) drug, df(2) = 2:

$$al_O = 10^{(pK - pH_O)} \qquad al_N = 10^{(pK - pH_N)}$$

(V.21)

The fractions of drug unionized, f_{ui}, are then given in both cases by the following equations:

$$f_{ui,O} = 1 - 1/(1 + al_O)$$

$$f_{ui,N} = 1 - 1/(1 + al_N)$$

(V.22)

Empirically derived expressions for the changes in df(3) and df(5), which appropriately limit the extent of change, are as follows:

$$df(3)_N = df(3)_O \cdot (3 + f_{ui,N})/(3 + f_{ui,O})$$

$$df(5)_N = df(5)_O \cdot (3 + f_{ui,N})/(3 + f_{ui,O})$$

(V.23)

8.2 Urine flow rate and pH, diuresis

For the standard subject the urine flow rate, sf(7), has a value of 0.066 l/h. This value may be raised to 0.2 l/h, to simulate the effect of dosage with a diuretic.

The urine pH, sf(8), has a value of 5.5 for the standard subject. Since it is the ionized form of a drug which is more rapidly excreted in the urine, raising the urine pH, e.g. by dosing with sodium bicarbonate, would be expected to increase the rate of excretion of a weakly acidic drug. Lowering the pH by dosing with ammonium chloride should increase the rate of excretion of a weakly basic drug.

The effects of changes in pH are treated in a similar manner to that used in Section 8.1 to describe the effect of pH changes on drug absorption. The fraction ionized, $f_i = 1 - f_{ui}$, is now used:

$$f_{i,O} = 1 - f_{ui,O} = 1/(1 + al_O)$$

$$f_{i,N} = 1 - f_{ui,N} = 1/(1 + al_N)$$

(V.24)

The change in pH governs change in the renal tubular function, df(14), for the drug according to an empirical expression. An increase in f_i leads to an increased rate of excretion, described in the model by a decrease in df(14).

$$df(14)_N = df(14)_O \cdot (1 + f_{i,O})/(1 + f_{i,N})$$

(V.25)

Increase of pH has a marked effect on the excretion of paracetamol, a very weak acid. The effect with the stronger salicylic acid is less marked. However, in cases of self-poisoning by aspirin overdose, the pH of the urine is likely to be below 5.5 and so this value should be set lower before the increase in pH brought about by bicarbonate dosing is introduced.

8.3 Enzyme induction

df(13) is a first-order rate constant for enzyme induction which acts to increase df(10), or df(11) in the case of saturable metabolism. Enzyme induction is a very slow process, taking many days of continued dosing to have an appreciable effect. df(13) is therefore small and is expressed in kilohour^{-1} (1 kh^{-1} = 0.001 h^{-1}, corresponding to a half-life of $0.693/0.001 = 693$ h or nearly 29 days).

Enzyme induction is seen particularly with carbamazepine and with phenobarbitone. When repeated doses of these drugs are given over several weeks, the mean steady-state plasma concentration begins to decrease due to the higher rate of metabolism arising from the enzyme induction.

8.4 Drug factors relating directly to plasma levels

Four drug factors are directly related to plasma levels: df(16), df(17), df(18) and df(19).

df(16) is the minimum plasma concentration for toxicity expressed in mg/l; when the set value is exceeded, the message 'toxicity' is printed out in the table of results. In the graphs this minimum toxic level is shown by a full horizontal line.

df(17) is the lethal drug concentration; when exceeded the calculations are stopped and an explanatory message is output.

df(18) is the minimum plasma concentration for drug activity, shown by a broken horizontal line on the graphs; when plasma levels are below this value the symbol '−' is printed in the table of results. When the level is exceeded but is below the mean of df(16) and df(18), the symbol printed is '+'; when the level exceeds this mean but is below df(18), the symbol '++' is printed.

df(19) specifies the units to be used for the graphs and tables of plasma concentrations. For the drugs currently available in the simulation, two sets of units have been found to be adequate; df(19) = 1 gives plasma concentrations in mg/l; df(19) = 2 gives them in μg/l.

Setting up a New Drug Using an Extra Drug File

1. PRELIMINARY EVALUATION OF THE DRUG FACTORS

The 18 effective drug factors may be divided into four groups as follows:

(i)   those which may be set up directly from published values or which are not not required for a particular drug;
(ii)   those evaluated from experimental data following i.v. dose;
(iii) those found from oral data;
(iv)   those found from i.m. data.

With some drugs, data following i.v. injection may not be available, in such cases the main evaluation has to be made using experimental results following dose by the oral or by the i.m. route.

When the oral or the i.m. route is not used, the drug factors associated with this route are all set to zero.

1.1 Factors set up directly

Valuable sources of information on physical and pharmacokinetic properties of many drugs are Martindale (*The Extra Pharmacopoeia*) and Clarke's *Isolation and Identification of Drugs* (see bibliography).

$df(1)$: the pK_a value is found from the literature.

$df(2)$: the acid–base index goes with the pK_a and is defined by the way in which the drug ionizes.

$df(6)$: the spare factor is given the value zero for all drugs.

$df(7)$: the fraction bound to plasma protein at therapeutic concentrations can generally be found from Clarke or from the summary of the literature on the drug in Martindale, alternatively it is obtained from review article(s) on the drug.

$df(9)$: the distribution ratio determines the apparent volume of distribution of the drug. Estimates of this volume may usually be found in reviews of the pharmacokinetics of the drug, references to which are given in Martindale. Values for many drugs in l/(kg body mass) are given in Clarke.

It is advantageous to define df(9) before runs to simulate experimental data are made. Study of the drugs in the program indicates that as a rough guide, 1 unit of df(9) is equivalent to about 60 l of apparent distribution volume in the standard subject, though some drugs show wide variation. As a start, the value of df(9) may be reckoned by dividing the apparent volume of distribution for a 70-kg subject found from the literature by 60. This first estimate may need to be altered subsequently.

df(13): the enzyme induction rate constant is only required for the few drugs which are known to induce their own metabolism. This factor is expressed in units of kilohour^{-1}, phenobarbitone is given the value 1.0. Non-inducing drugs are given the value zero.

df(16): the minimum plasma level for toxic effects may usually be found from Martindale, from Clarke or from reviews, as can df(17), the lethal plasma level, and df(18), the minimum level for drug activity. There is an extensive table of values of these three parameters in a paper by A.H.Stead and A.C.Moffat [*Hum. Toxicol.*, (1983) **3**, 437–464].

df(19): an administrative factor which determines the concentration units for output in tables or graphs. If df(19) equals 1, the units are mg/l and if df(19) equals 2, the units are µg/litre. These two sets have been found adequate for all the drugs so far considered.

1.2 General considerations for setting up factors from experimental data

To start the process of setting values for the other factors, values for a drug with properties similar to those of the one under study are examined and preliminary values for the new one are decided. The factors for all the drugs on the main list of the simulation program are given in Appendix IV.

1.3 Setting up the preliminary drug file

When a preliminary set of factors has been decided, a new drug file is set up. The file name is limited to eight letters and so it may be the name of the drug or the first eight letters of this name if it is a long one.

The file consists of three lines in the format as set out in Appendix IV for the main list drugs in the program. The first line is the full drug name, with 16 spaces available; the second contains the values of df(1)–df(10) each with a space after the number, decimal points are required for each number, including zero; the third line consists of df(11)–df(19) plus the two lag times, set out in the same format as the second line. Both the lag times may be set to zero if required.

On entering the simulation program, the new drug file may be accessed by first pressing <ENTER> alone when asked for the choice of drug, as described in Chapter 4, Section 2, and then specifying the drug file name.

When experimental plasma concentrations following i.v. dose are available, the preliminary values for the factors are set up and runs then made, prescribing the new drug, to simulate the experimental data. The factors are further altered in the light of the results obtained, until a reasonable fit between experimental and simulated data is obtained.

The process is then repeated with oral and i.m. data as available, to give a complete set of factors for the new drug. The drug file may be edited to incorporate the improved parameters as they are determined.

When i.v. data are not available, the factor evaluation has to be based on oral and/or i.m. data.

In the simplified metabolism scheme used in the simulation program, 'drug' means unchanged drug plus any active metabolites, while 'metabolite' means all the inactive metabolites formed.

2. FINDING AND EVALUATING FACTORS

2.1 Factors found from i.v. experimental data

Ideally these data should consist of experimental measurements of plasma concentrations at a series of times after i.v. bolus injection, including short times. In addition, there should be information on the total excretion of the unchanged drug and its metabolites. Unfortunately, with some drugs i.v. data are not available.

The parameters to be estimated are df(8), the distribution rate constant; df(10), or df(11) and df(12), the metabolism rate constants; and df(14), the renal tubular function.

The early part of the C,t plot is governed mainly by distribution and metabolism, while in the later part metabolism and urinary excretion are the main factors.

df(8). If the $\log(C),t$ plot is linear for all except the first point or two, the complete volume of distribution is rapidly reached and df(8) may be given a relatively high value; if the plot has more prolonged curvature, the final volume of distribution is reached more slowly and a value of 1 h^{-1} or less may be given to df(8) as a starting value.

df(10), df(11), df(12). The metabolic rate constants depend on whether the metabolism is first-order or capacity limited; in the first case, df(11) and df(12) are set to zero and df(10) is given a preliminary value; in the second case, df(10) is set to zero and values are required for df(11) and df(12). Starting values may sometimes be established from published kinetic studies with the drug.

df(14). The renal tubular function, df(14), governs the rate of urinary excretion of unchanged drug. If the drug is mainly excreted unchanged it has a low value, say 0.2–2; when little drug is excreted unchanged, much higher values are used.

The distribution, metabolism and excretion factors are adjusted to give the correct half-life of the drug in the linear part of the $\log(C),t$ plot. The factors are balanced to give the correct ratio of total excretion of unchanged drug to total amount metabolized. Remember that in the simplified metabolic scheme used in MuPharm, 'drug' means original drug plus active metabolites and 'metabolite' means all the inactive metabolites.

2.2 Factors to be evaluated from oral dose data

If i.v. data are available and have been used to develop drug factors as described above, we can proceed to study kinetic data following oral dose of the drug. The factors to be evaluated are df(3), the rate constant for absorption from the GIT, and df(5), the fraction absorbed from an oral dose.

df(3). df(3) governs the shape of the early part of the C,t plot. When the maximum concentration occurs within an hour or less of dose, then absorption is rapid and df(3) may be given a high starting value, say 2 h^{-1}; when the peak concentration occurs at several hours after dose, df(3) should be given an initial value of 0.1 h^{-1} or less.

When i.v. data are available it is usually not too difficult to evaluate the oral dose parameters. However, sometimes the factor values derived from i.v. data may have to be modified as a result of oral dose results. In such cases compromise values between i.v. and oral routes have to be decided upon.

When i.v. data are not available, there is the more difficult job of fitting all the factors so far discussed — distribution, metabolism, excretion and absorption — from the oral data.

L. Saunders, D. Ingram and S. H. D. Jackson

2.3 Factors from i.m. data

df(4). df(4) is the rate constant for absorption from an i.m. deposit.

df(15). df(15) is the fraction of the i.m. dose taken up into the plasma. This fraction is generally near to 1.0 but there are exceptions, see Chapter 1, Section 8.3.

These two factors are evaluated from experimental i.m. dose data in a similar way to that used for the oral factors.

If the i.m. route is not used for the drug under consideration, both the factors are set to zero.

3. LAG TIMES

In addition to the 19 drug factors, lag times for oral and i.m. routes must be specified. These lag times are properties of the preparation rather than of the drug itself and in the drug file they may both be set to zero. Alternatively they may be given values for usual preparations of the drug. These values may be assessed from early time C,t data as in Chapter 1, Section 8.2.

4. AN EXAMPLE: SETTING UP FACTORS FOR CARBAMAZEPINE

The literature references used are the section on carbamazepine in Martindale and the paper by Palmer, Bertilsson, Collste and Rawlins [*Clin. Pharmacol. Ther.*, (1973) **14**, 827–832], which gives details of plasma concentrations following oral dose.

Carbamazepine is a tricyclic substance, analogous in chemical structure to nortriptyline. df(1) and df(2) have the values 9 and 2 respectively; df(6), as for all drugs, is zero.

df(7): the fraction bound to plasma protein is reported as 0.73.

df(9): the distribution ratio is assessed from a reported mean distribution volume of 1.3 l/kg; for the standard subject, the volume will be 70×1.3 l and when this is divided by 60, the resulting provisional value for df(9) is 1.5.

There is evidence of quite rapid enzyme induction and so df(13) is given a value of 2 kh^{-1}, twice the value for phenobarbitone.

df(16): df(16) the minimum toxic level, is set to 10 mg/l; df(17), the lethal level, is set to 40 mg/l; df(18), the minimum active level is 4 mg/l; df(19), the concentration unit factor is set to 1 (for mg/l).

Preliminary values for the other factors are assessed as follows.

df(3): gastro-intestinal absorption is reported to be slow and so this factor is given the value 0.1 h^{-1}; the i.m. route is not normally used and so *df(4)* and *df(15)* are set to 0.

df(5): the drug is almost completely absorbed from an oral dose so the fraction absorbed is given the value 1.0.

The rate of distribution, df(8), is given a presumed value of 2 h^{-1}.

Carbamazepine is extensively metabolized and there is no evidence of limited-capacity effects. df(10) is set to 2 h^{-1}; df(11) and df(12) are consequently given values of zero.

The drug is excreted almost entirely as metabolite and so the renal tubular function, df(14), is set at a relatively high value of 20 so as to limit the urinary excretion of unchanged drug.

In the absence of detailed experimental information, the two lag times are both set to zero.

The set of preliminary factors is now complete and the drug file may be set up.

```
carbamazepine

9. 2. 0.1 0. 1. 0. .73 2. 1.5 2.

0. 0. 2. 20. 0. 10. 40. 4. 1. 0. 0.
```

Matching of the simulated results with experimental data on plasma levels, on change of half-life with continued dosing and on urinary excretion produces the following modifications:

```
df(3) = 0.05; df(8) = 1.0; df(9) = 1.7; df(10) = 0.44;
df(13) = 1.5; df(14) = 18.
```

The drug file is then re-edited to put in these values and is almost ready for use. Suitable runs should now be made to compare plasma half-life, area under the C,t curve, apparent volume of distribution and total clearance with the information on carbamazepine given in Clarke's *Isolation and Identification of Drugs*.

All drug factor files should be regarded as tentative and may need to be modified in the light of further information on the drug.

Creating a Preset Subject Using an Extra Subject File

Extra files may be set up containing details of different subjects in the same way as for extra drugs. The file is set up outside the simulation program and is called by pressing <ENTER> alone at the dialogue question on choice of subject (Chapter 4, Section 3.3).

The file name is limited to eight characters and the file consists of three lines. The first line has 40 spaces available for a brief description of the subject. The second line contains the four subject characteristics: height (cm), mass (kg), age (years) and sex, 1 for male, 2 for female; it should consist just of the four numbers with spaces between them, each number being given a decimal point. The third line consists of the nine factors for the subject, again as numbers with decimal points, separated by spaces.

The nine normal factors for the subject are found by entering the simulation program, making a prescription of any drug and entering the run details and then the four characteristics — height, mass, age and sex — for this subject. The CHANGE sub-menu is then chosen and option 3, change subject factors, is selected. The screen then shows the current values of all the normal factors for this subject.

It is necessary to enter all nine factors into line 3 of the subject file even when they are not changed from those shown on the screen. They can be rounded to three significant figures. The advantage of this arrangement is that any of the factors [except preferably sf(5)] can be modified for the extra subject file. For example, a hepatic dysfunction may be given by reducing sf(6); a renal dysfunction may be given by reducing sf(9).

Example

As an example of setting up an extra subject file, consider a 55-year-old female, height 152 cm, mass 62 kg, with a 40% loss of hepatic function.

The first step is to enter the simulation program and prescribe say 500 mg of ampicillin, oral; run length 4 h, four results at 1-h intervals; choose own subject and enter the above characteristics. Then choose CHANGE and change subject factors and note down the values of the nine subject factors, altering sf(6) to 0.6. There is no need to make the run.

Now come out of the simulation program and set up the subject file, which we give the name SUBJ3HD.

```
Subject3;55y,female,hepatic function0.6

152. 62. 55. 2.

2.01 16. 3.5 36.4 .646 .6 .036 5. 3.62
```

The first line is a title and a brief summary of the subject, limited to 40 spaces; the second line gives the four main characteristics; the third line is taken from the screen display of subject factors, with factor 6 altered to 0.6.

The file is now ready for loading in a subsequent simulation run.

Changing the Iteration Interval

The iteration interval, t_I, for the calculations is set at a normal value of 0.01 h and remains unchanged throughout a run.

The real time taken to complete a run is inversely proportional to t_I; very long runs may be speeded up by increasing it to 0.02 h, but further increase may cause instability in the calculations. If this instability occurs, a message is printed out recommending reduction in t_I.

The value of t_I may be used to control the speed at which the disposition diagram changes (Chapter 2, Section 4.3).

Table VIII.1 shows the results for a short run with 400 mg of phenytoin given to the standard subject by the oral route. This prescription is chosen because the absorption of phenytoin is quite slow, giving plasma concentrations which are changing continuously over several hours. The run time is 4 h with results every 0.25 h.

Column headings are time, then iteration intervals in h, the last column shows the percent divergence between the concentration values for the smallest and the largest iteration interval.

The calculated concentrations are in mg/l.

It is seen that the results agree to within 1.4% at 1 h and then converge further at later times. With very short runs where the early results are important, as with the anaesthetic thiopentone, reduction of the iteration interval improves the precision of the calculations but increases the time required to execute them.

Table VIII.1 Phenytoin 400 mg oral; standard subject.

Time (h)	0.0001	0.001	0.005	0.01	0.02	% div
0.25	2.24	2.25	2.28	2.31	2.42	7.4
0.5	3.42	3.42	3.44	3.46	3.51	2.6
0.75	4.37	4.37	4.39	4.41	4.49	2.7
1.0	5.16	5.16	5.17	5.19	5.23	1.4
1.5	6.34	6.34	6.36	6.37	6.40	1.0
2.0	7.14	7.14	7.15	7.16	7.19	0.7
3.0	7.99	7.99	8.00	8.00	8.02	0.4
4.0	8.29	8.29	8.29	8.29	8.30	0.1

Table VIII.2 Thiopentone 250 mg i.v. bolus; standard subject.

Time (h)	0.0001	0.001	0.005	0.01	% div
0.02	55.49	55.99	58.36	61.63	11.1
0.04	44.26	44.61	46.26	48.51	9.6
0.07	31.51	31.71	32.62	33.84	7.4
0.1	22.46	22.56	23.02	23.62	5.2
0.14	14.41	14.44	14.57	14.72	2.2
0.17	10.45	10.45	10.46	10.45	0.0
0.2	7.71	7.70	7.64	7.56	-1.9
0.25	4.91	4.89	4.81	4.70	-4.2
0.3	3.43	3.42	3.35	3.26	-5.0
0.35	2.66	2.65	2.60	2.54	-4.5
0.4	2.25	2.25	2.22	2.18	-3.1
0.5	1.93	1.93	1.92	1.91	-1.0

In Table VIII.2, the results of a series of runs with different values of t_1 are given, for a 0.5-h run with 250 mg of thiopentone given as an i.v. bolus to the standard subject. Thiopentone is chosen because the plasma concentrations are changing rapidly over a short time interval.

The headings of the columns are time, followed by values of t_1 in h, the last column shows the percentage divergence between results with iteration intervals of 0.01 and 0.0001 h.

The concentrations are in mg/l.

The divergences are large and positive at first then pass through zero at 0.17 h and become negative, eventually decreasing to -1% at 0.5 h.

This searching test of the variation of the calculated C values with iteration interval shows that for an unusual run of this type, there is an advantage in reducing the value of t_1 to say 0.001 h.

Answers to Problems

Chapter 2

1.

Area	Ampicillin	Theophylline
trapezia	21.14	67.80
extrapolation	0.24	3.62
total	21.38 mg h/l	71.42 mg h/l

2. Oxprenolol
$k = 0.411 \text{ h}^{-1}$, $t_{1/2} = 1.69$ h, area = 0.848 h mg/l. $Cl_T = 23.6$, $Cl_r = 0.006$, $Cl_h = 23.6$ l/h; $V = 57.4$ l.

Chapter 3

1. Oxprenolol, zero lag time, C_{max} 456 µg/l at 0.75h. $k = 0.379 \text{ h}^{-1}$, $t_{1/2} = 1.83$ h, area = 2.00 h mg/l. $F = 0.590$, $F_a = 1.0$, $E = 0.410$.
2. Amoxycillin, parameters similar to ampicillin except that for oral dose, C_{max} is doubled, $F = 0.964$, $F_a = 1.0$, $E = 0.036$.
3. Phenobarbitone, $C_{max} = 8.1$ mg/l at 3.5 h, $t_{lag} = 0$. i.m., $k = 0.0079 \text{ h}^{-1}$, $t_{1/2} = 87.8$h, area = 1124 h mg/l, 100 mg/0.5 h i.v., area = 395 h mg/l, $Cl_T = 0.25$ l/h, $V = 32.0$ l, $F = 0.95$.

Chapter 5

1. Theophylline, for a target of 15 mg/l, 42 mg/h, 500-mg over 2 h, loading dose.
2. Benzylpenicillin, 1600 mg every 2 h gives steady-state peak of 96.3 mg/l.
3. Phenobarbitone, 75 mg every 24 h, 450-mg loading dose.

Chapter 6

1. Indomethacin, $Cl_T = 4.91$ l/h, $V = 69.8$ l, $F = 0.927$.
   Regimen with conventional dose, 50 mg every 8 h.
   Regimen with sustained release, 120 mg every 12 h.
2. Gentamicin, target 6 mg/l, 160 mg i.m. every 6 h.

Chapter 7

1. Aspirin (12 h runs):

Dose (mg)	Area (mg h/l)	Dose/area ratio (l/h)	$t_{1/2}$ (h)
500	109	4.59	2.21
2000	981	2.04	4.34
5000	5935	0.93	12.9

$F = 0.80$, $V = 11.9$ l.

2. Aspirin, assuming first-order kinetics, 3000 mg oral every 6 h, rapidly reaches toxic levels. 1050 mg oral every 6 h, loading dose 3500 mg.

Chapter 8

1.

Dysfunction	Oxprenolol	Atenolol
hepatic	higher C and $t_{1/2}$	no effect
renal	no effect	higher C and $t_{1/2}$

Chapter 9

6.1 Gentamicin. (i) 100 mg, (ii) 7 h, (iii) 70 mg every 8 h, peak 8.22, trough 2.53 mg/l. Renal impairment, after 6th dose, peak 11.4, trough 5.6.

Dosing interval (h)	Peak (mg/l)	Trough (mg/l)
10	9.94	4.05
12	8.95	3.03
14	8.26	2.33

70 mg every 14 h is therefore suitable for this subject.

6.2   Theophylline. 180-mg dose, approximate steady state at 60 h, peak 6.9, trough 4.7 mg/l. 300-mg dose, steady state 60 h, peak 11.4, trough 7.8.

6.3   Lignocaine. (a) C falls below toxic level within 0.25 h. (b) 90 mg/h (1.5 mg/min), $C = 4.3$ mg/l at 9 h. (c) 150 mg/0.02 h is suitable loading dose, gives active levels at 0.1 h.

6.4   Digoxin.

| Serum creatinine | mg/l after 7th dose | |
(mmol/l)	peak	Trough
0.1	2.23	1.07
0.15	2.58	1.38
0.2	2.81	1.60
0.25	2.97	1.75

At a serum creatinine of 0.2 mmol/litre, the peak exceeds the toxic level and so the dose should be reduced.

When the serum creatinine stabilizes at 0.25 mmol/l a regimen of 0.0625 mg every 24 h with a loading dose of 0.5 mg gives after the 7th dose, peak = 1.78, trough = 1.14 mg/l. After 14 doses the results are peak = 1.82, trough = 1.18. This regimen is therefore satisfactory.

Bibliography

larke's Isolation and Identification of Drugs, 2nd edn (1986). The Pharmaceutical Press, London.

.Clarke and D.A.Smith, *An Introduction to Pharmacokinetics*, 2nd edn (1986). Blackwell Scientific, Oxford.

.H.Curry, *Drug Disposition and Kinetics*, 3rd edn (1980). Blackwell Scientific, Oxford.

1.Gibaldi and D.Perrier, *Pharmacokinetics*, Vol. 15 of *Drugs and the Pharmaceutical Sciences* (1982). Marcel Dekker, New York.

1.Gibaldi, *Biopharmaceutics and Clinical Pharmacokinetics*, 3rd edn (1984). Lea and Febiger, Philadelphia.

).G.Grahame-Smith and J.K.Aronson, *The Oxford Textbook of Clinical Pharmacology and Drug Therapy* (1984). Oxford University Press, Oxford.

Martindale, *The Extra Pharmacopoeia*, 28th edn (1982). The Pharmaceutical Press, London.

.E.Notari, *Biopharmaceutics and Clinical Pharmacokinetics*, 4th edn (1987). Marcel Dekker, New York.

1.Rowland and D.Tozer, *Clinical Pharmacokinetics* (1980). Lea and Febiger, Philadelphia.

'.Turner and A.Richens, *Clinical Pharmacology*, 4th edn (1982). Churchill Livingstone, Edinburgh.

Index